IN THE ICY GRIP OF
FEAR...

What had started as a pleasant swim had now become an adventure of exploration. As I swam onward, I had to thread my way among tall, waving kelp beds. But ahead the kelp was parted as though by some current, forming a tunnel through which I could swim. It was dark in here, and I began to be nervous and then frightened as darkness closed in about me. Then, suddenly, the kelp was gone, but there was no relief from the darkness or the sense of confinement. And then my reaching hand touched stone, and, shuddering, I realized I had entered a natural underwater tunnel into a world of complete darkness—a world of terror! I wanted to scream and turn back, but I couldn't. For I was already trapped. . . .

Sinister House

by
Caroline Farr

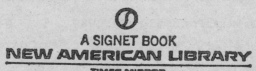

A SIGNET BOOK
NEW AMERICAN LIBRARY
TIMES MIRROR
in association with Horwitz Publications

SIGNET TRADEMARK REG. U.S. PAT. OFF. AND FOREIGN COUNTRIES
REGISTERED TRADEMARK—MARCA REGISTRADA
HECHO EN CHICAGO, U.S.A.

SIGNET, SIGNET CLASSICS, MENTOR, PLUME AND MERIDIAN BOOKS
are published by The New American Library, Inc.,
1301 Avenue of the Americas, New York, New York 10019

FIRST SIGNET PRINTING, JANUARY, 1978

1 2 3 4 5 6 7 8 9

PRINTED IN THE UNITED STATES OF AMERICA

Sinister House

1

Paul Acton and I started dating in the spring of 1974 when we met while watching a political demonstration with which we both disagreed. Paul was twenty-four and completing his final year at law school. I was twenty-one and in my senior year of college, which was as far as I expected to go on the scholarship I'd won at high school. Paul had his academic future in law worked out to the last detail, but I couldn't make up my mind whether I wanted to teach or become a librarian.

I guess we were opposites in lots of other ways, too. I'm small with black hair and dark blue eyes. Paul's blond, gray-eyed, and handsome, with an athlete's wide shoulders and flat stomach he earned playing halfback at Stanford. The only sport I've ever been any good at is swimming.

I think I fell in love with Paul the first time he took me out. It seemed incredible to me that he even wanted to. Why should he, when half the glamorous types on the campus would have come running if he whistled . . . well, almost? He was one of those men who attract women without even trying. And the fact that the Actons were one of the wealthiest families in California and his mother, Vanessa, was continually mentioned in the social columns had nothing to do with it. Any girl on campus would have told you she could fall for someone like Paul even if all he had was the scholarship he was battling his way through college with.

At first Paul used to take other girls out too; then after our fourth or fifth date, he seemed to lose interest and dated only me. By then, although I tried to hide it, I think I realized my case was hopeless. Not that our social life together was all that exciting, or even a pale shadow of his mother's, but that was the way we both liked it.

We just went to low-key coffee houses, like Menhuins' in Palo Alto, or to the New Life, a downtown disco that was his favorite place. On one special occasion, my birthday, he borrowed a friend's car, because he didn't have one of his own, and drove me to Fisherman's Wharf for a fabulous seafood dinner. And of course, when Paul played football and I could afford a ticket, or Paul could scrounge a complimentary pass, I was his most ardent fan. Luckily for my blood pressure, the season was almost over when I met Paul. All three times I watched, he was the star of the game, and the result was a cliffhanger.

We were in Menhuins' coffee house when he

made the remark that was to change my life. "Samantha," he said, "what about our marriage?"

I almost choked on a piece of chocolate cake. "What marriage?" I gasped, making myself heard above the coffee-making and the conversation.

"Ours, of course." Momentarily I thought he looked as surprised by what he had said as I had been to hear it.

I was in love with Paul Acton, but it hadn't occurred to me that Paul might have fallen in love in return. A girl can dream, but this was reality. I could tell he meant it.

"You want me to . . . *marry* you?"

"Yes."

"But why?" I gasped. "I mean . . ." I stopped, because right then I didn't know what I meant.

"*Why?*" His brows drew together, and he looked uneasy and puzzled. "All I can say is, why the hell do you think I've been hanging around for months unless I had something like that in mind?"

"I thought you might just want to seduce me," I ventured.

"That too," he said. "But *not* as the end result. I like you, Samantha, I like you very much. And . . . you like me. . . . Well, don't you?"

"Yes . . ." I admitted.

"Then we like each other. So now, will you marry me?"

"I suppose that's a good reason . . . ?"

"In fact, for my part, I love you, Samantha."

I told him that was a better reason, and he kissed me across the table, to the interest of some of the other customers, who encouraged him with uncouth remarks.

When I came down off cloud nine, I realized I was out in the night air and we were walking toward the bus stop.

"Vanessa is staying at the St. Francis for the weekend," he was telling me. "You'll have to meet Vanessa. You'll like her, I hope. She can be a very sweet person when she wants."

"Vanessa?" I demanded suspiciously. "You mean your mother?"

"Yes, of course, my mother. I always call her Vanessa, she likes it that way, and most of the time she looks too young for the part, anyway."

The Vanessa Acton of the social columns, the heiress to the Acton wealth, I was thinking in sudden dismay. *That* Vanessa! The thought of meeting her as Paul's fiancée was sending cold shivers down my spine.

"Look, why don't we grab a cab and go over there now?" he suggested with appalling enthusiasm. "Maybe she won't *be* there yet. She was flying from Los Angeles and driving here from the airport. But we can wait in the hotel. I'll buy you a drink! What do you say, Samantha?"

I stared down at myself in horror. "Meet your mother wearing *jeans*? At the St. Francis? You have to be joking!"

"But you look great in jeans," he said.

"No, Paul!"

"Maybe you're right," he conceded slowly. "Tomorrow afternoon, then? That's when she's expecting to see me. Hey, wear that dress you wore to dinner on your birthday! The red one! Will you?"

"Well . . ." I said, pretending. "If that's what you want Paul." It was the best dress I had to go to a place like the St. Francis on a Saturday afternoon, anyhow. I had already decided on it.

"Great!" he said. He hesitated. "Samantha?"

"Yes?"

"About the ring . . ."

"Ring?" I puzzled.

"A guy usually gives a girl a ring when she promises to marry him."

"Did I say that?" I asked, really startled by the possibility of marriage looming for the first time.

"If you didn't mean yes, why did you kiss me?" he demanded with typical male logic.

"So okay. I meant yes."

We had stopped a few yards from the commuters waiting at the bus stop. They looked half asleep, but when he kissed me again, they seemed to wake up.

"That brings us back to the ring, doesn't it?" he said when I made him release me, and came back down off my tiptoes.

"Ring?" He'd left me behind.

"We'll buy one in the morning, Samantha," he said eagerly. "But there's something you have to know about me first."

Oh, no! Did he already have a wife, or a fi-

ancée, the Bluebeard? Luckily, he didn't wait
for me to answer.

"My father was accidentally killed," he said,
trying to get it all out quickly, because the bus
was coming. "The only will he left was made
when I was in grade school. It left me an annu-
ity to put me through Stanford. It's like your
scholarship, pays barely enough, with the current inflation, to pay my study costs and living
expenses at Stanford. . . ." He hesitated,
embarrassed.

"Mine doesn't even do that," I told him.
"That's why I have to work. But go on, Paul."

"What I mean is . . . it won't be the kind
of ring I'd like to buy you, Samantha. But
maybe later . . ."

"It will be a beautiful ring, Paul," I told him.
"I'll love it, I know." Because he showed signs
of wanting to kiss me again, I added hastily,
"The bus is coming!"

"Dad meant to make another will," he said,
coming back to earth. "Vanessa controls everything now. I have to rely on an allowance from
her, as I had to rely on Dad when he was alive.
That was okay in past years, so I didn't bother
Dad then, or Vanessa."

"We can build our own marriage, Paul."

He nodded. The bus was pulling in. "I
wanted you to say that, Samantha! Because
that's what I want to do. I've never worked
harder than I have since we met. I think I've
known all the time just what I wanted to do,
and I've done it. I'm going to pass, and I'm going to be close to the top—you'll see! And then,

you just watch those offers come in from the
law firms! And the day we accept the best offer,
we can marry."

The bus pulled in then, to the disappointment of the listeners.

Back in my tiny apartment with the door
closed and Paul on his way home to the larger
apartment he shared with a roommate, I came
back slowly to earth and looked at myself in
the mirror. I *looked* the same. A little flushed,
but that was from Paul's good-night kiss on
the steps outside the apartment house. We
were not allowed male visitors beyond that
point. But here I was, engaged to marry Paul
Acton!

And about to meet his mother, Vanessa Acton, for the first time tomorrow. I rushed to get
out my red dress, and examined it anxiously. It
looked ordinary, I decided. But perhaps if I left
the neck open and wore it with the red-and-
beige print scarf Paul bought me for my birthday . . .

I met Paul in town on the corner near the
jeweler's, and there wasn't much choice in diamonds in our price range. Fortunately, the jeweler was used to people with little money to
spend. After all, it was a college town. So he
found one for us. He admitted that the stone in
the center had a flaw. It was no giant, either,
but it was larger than most of the others at the
same price, and Paul determined that the dia-
mond chips surrounding it looked *great*.

I didn't comment. I'd never had an engage-

ment ring before, and Paul was buying it for
me. *I loved it.* I told Paul I'd never want another, no matter how much money he made
when he became an attorney.

In the taxi taking us to the St. Francis, I began to get stage fright again at the thought of
meeting Paul's mother. And Paul seemed almost as nervous as I was, though he kept reassuring me everything was going to be fine. I
wanted to run away when the familiar facade
of the St. Francis came in sight. Familiar, I
mean, because I'd often passed it and wondered what kind of people stayed there. Paul
wouldn't agree when, terrified, I suggested
maybe it would be better if we left it for a few
weeks, or maybe months, until Vanessa got
more used to the idea of meeting me.

"Or vice versa?" Paul suggested ironically,
adding, "Samantha, she isn't going to *eat* you!"

"Then why are *you* so scared?" I asked him,
shaking.

"Who's scared?" he demanded, fumbling nervously for his billfold as the taxi stopped with a
flourish at the foot of marble steps, and a doorman in a gilt-trimmed uniform came down to
open the door for me.

"Look! Let's be reasonable!" I mumbled,
drawing back from the opening door. "We can
always come back another time, when we get
more used to the idea!"

"Samantha, please!" he said. "Let's get this
thing over, and . . ." He broke off abruptly.
"Uhuh! Too late! Don't look now, but we've got

a one-woman welcoming committee waiting at the top of the steps."

He was right. I couldn't mistake the woman standing up there. I had seen her picture too often in the glossy women's magazines since I started going out with Paul, and learned that she was his mother. And besides, she had Paul's good looks and the same thick blond hair that shone in the afternoon sun. The only difference I could note, as I forced my trembling legs not to run away in the other direction, was that her eyes were brown. Large and brown and Latin, the ones God should've given me to go with my black hair, instead of ones that were Irish violet.

"Hi there," she said, studying my nervous approach.

"Hi," I ventured. Hers sounded about the way I imagined someone would say "Hi there" if she were from Boston and upper class—the tone didn't suit the words.

"I saw you coming. I was sitting in the lounge," she said. "You're late, Paul. Shall we go inside?"

"Sorry, Vanessa," Paul said. "We were delayed coming over." He was ushering us inside while the doorman held open the door. I tried to hang back, but Vanessa politely made that impossible by following *me*. Walking into a lounge over deep carpet, with me plotting a course between potted palms, I could feel Vanessa's eyes studying me with clinical efficiency from behind. My hair, my waist, I felt them explore more slowly down to the hemline and lower still to the backs of my legs.

"I like your dress," she said, drawing up beside me.

"Thank you." Should I call her Mrs. Acton, or wait till Paul introduced us? I settled for the wait.

"It's very nice," she said. And added speculatively, "It suits your coloring."

"Thank you." She could also have told me, I was sure, how much, or rather how little, it cost.

"You're very attractive," she added as a bonus. "There's a little lounge on the left, where it's more private. Turn here. You've had lunch?"

"Yes, thank you." That *was* the object of the exercise, that we come after lunch. I hoped Paul was following, that he hadn't deserted me—but I was afraid to look back, in case he had.

"It's rather a shock to be informed that your son intends to marry, and you realize he isn't a boy anymore."

"It must be!" I muttered. After all, she'd only had twenty-four years to get used to the idea that Paul was growing up.

"I'm glad you understand," she said.

"Oh, perfectly." I understood, all right, all right! I understood and recognized the resentment beneath that smooth talk. Resentment against my intrusion upon what she considered a perfect relationship between mother and son. I sensed she hated girls like me, students who might try to take Paul away from her. Right then I could have returned the compliment. But Paul had followed me into the poky little lounge.

"Can I get you a drink, Vanessa?"

"No. But if you press the button over there, someone will come to take the order, and charge it to me." She studied me speculatively. "What would you like?"

"Could I have some orange juice, please?" I decided quickly.

"But of course. Paul?"

"I'll have bourbon, and water."

A waiter appeared like a genie in answer to Paul's ring. We sat down stiffly as she reminded Paul, "Don't I get introduced to your fiancée, young man?"

"Of course!" he mumbled. "This is Samantha, Mother—the girl I told you I intend to marry. Samantha, this is my mother."

"Samantha?" She gave him an inquiring look.

"Samantha *Walton*, Mother."

"There were Waltons who had a beach house near Finisterre."

"Not the same," he said shortly. "Samantha lives in Palo Alto."

"Ah," she said. "How d'you do, Samantha."

"How d'you do, Mrs. Acton."

"You're a student?"

"Yes, I'm an English major."

"Ah," she said. "Do you intend to use your degree, if you get it? Or do you mean to make a profession of marriage?"

I said, "I mean to use it; Paul and I have to

make a home." And if she thought I was marrying Paul because *she* was the Acton millionairess and Paul was her son, maybe *that* would show her how wrong she was.

It didn't.

"How soon do you propose to marry Paul?" she asked coldly, as though Paul wasn't a party to what we intended.

I ventured a small smile, because in the circumstances, I found her question amusing. "I really don't know, Mrs. Acton. Paul only asked me yesterday. I'm still in a daze, I guess. And we both have to graduate."

For the first time she looked at me as though she had some hope for me. But not much.

"I think young people who rush into marriage are foolish," she declared dogmatically.

"I agree, Mrs. Acton."

That was the extent of our conversation. After that remark of mine, the things we said had no real meaning. Not until she looked at her watch and told Paul she'd almost forgotten she had a friend taking her out to dinner. We got up then at once and said good-bye politely. She went back to her room, and we walked back down the marble steps to where the doorman helped us into a taxi. And *I* breathed a deep sigh of relief.

"I tried to tell you it would be better to call her Vanessa," Paul said, leaning back as we drove away.

"Yeah, I know. But I preferred to call her Mrs. Acton. Besides, you don't call a woman that much older than you by her first name. Not unless she invites you to."

"Maybe next time?"

"Maybe."

He took my hand and held it and looked at me anxiously. "What do you think of her, Samantha?"

"She's beautiful, elegant, very fond of you of course; she's everything the social columns say about her."

"Samantha! I asked you what *you* think of my mother," he reminded me sternly.

"I think she doesn't like me."

"So you don't like her," he said glumly, looking his disappointment.

"I didn't say that, Paul," I told him, thinking about that. "I admire her. Any girl would. I *want* to like her. I'd like nothing better than to have your mother like me. I *want* to be able to call her Vanessa, the way you say she likes best. Because if I could, and she'd let me, that would mean we were friends."

He shook his head and grinned apologetically. "I love her," he said. "Vanessa's spoiled, she always has been, but I love her. She's jealous, too. I know that, Samantha. She's resented every girlfriend I've had, ever since I can remember." He shook his head. "You don't have that on your own."

"Oh, *great!*" I said indignantly. "And how many *have* you had her inspect for you, Don Juan?"

"None of your business." He chuckled.

"Three, if you must know! But you're the only one I told her I meant to marry."

I was in his arms on the back seat of the taxi; then suddenly he was kissing me.

"What do I have to swear on to convince you, Samantha?" he asked me in mock anger when we recovered our breath. "Look! Cross my heart, *I love you!* Can't you believe that?"

"I believe it," I admitted. "A woman knows these things. That's part of my loving you. That's why I *want* to marry you."

"Then you can believe this too, Samantha," he said in a low voice. "Anything my mother or anyone else feels about it doesn't matter. I intend to marry you, no matter what! *I swear it, Samantha!* With or without my mother's blessing. Without the things my father meant to be mine but his death deprived me of, if we have to. These things don't matter. We can do without them. We can make our own way. Agreed, Samantha?"

"Agreed!" I told him, feeling tears welling because of the way he was looking at me.

We drove back to my apartment, holding hands in silence. We parted there, because with the end of the academic year approaching, we both wanted to study.

I changed into my pajamas and robe and made a pot of coffee. While waiting for the coffee to percolate I chose the textbooks I would need. The battle to relax and study after one of the most exciting days of my life began.

Under the circumstances, it was a long and arduous battle.

I worked late and awakened far from my best—with a head full of cotton and eyes still tired from too much small print. I put the percolator on again and headed for the shower, beginning to remember that today was Sunday, so there were no classes, and that Paul and I had agreed to go out someplace this afternoon and to cram only this morning.

The shower felt wonderful. I was appreciating it, with my head thrown back, my mouth open and water pelting my tired body delightfully, when quite distinctly I heard the doorbell ring. Only the shower heard what I said! I can't think of anything worse than having to rush from the shower to answer the doorbell. There was one thing, though—in this apartment, you knew it couldn't be a man. The Methodist group that ran the apartment house saw to that.

I put my head out from between the curtains and yelled, "*Who is it?*"

Somebody outside said something; it was impossible to decide what. But logic suggested it had to be Anne Amberg. Anne had the next apartment, and we worked together in the Stanford library and were always borrowing or lending each other books. Anne had been studying late last night too, and we'd had coffee together in my place around two A.M.

"I'm coming!"

I grabbed the bath towel hastily. Anne probably wanted to borrow a book this morning. She knew her way around; all I had to do was let her in.

I padded, dripping, across from the bathroom, opened the door, and gasped. Paul's mother stood there, staring at me with disbelief and disapproval, about the way you'd study some unpleasant specimen you'd noticed for the first time in the veterinary laboratory. I stared right back, more shocked than she was.

She looked past me and said, "It is Samantha Walton, isn't it? Am I intruding?" Her eyes searched the rooms behind me through the open bathroom and bedroom doors as though looking for someone, before they came back to stare at me. Smartly dressed in a beige designer suit, her makeup perfect, not a hair out of place, she looked as she had at the hotel. Mrs. Vanessa Acton, straight from the social page.

"I thought you were . . ." I lost the words as I clutched my bath towel tighter around me. Under that sarcastic stare, it seemed to be shrinking.

"Paul, perhaps?" she inquired politely.

"We're not allowed male visitors."

"Really? I thought everything was coeducational these days." She frowned. "I came around for a little chat with you, Samantha. I phoned Paul and asked him to bring you to lunch, but he said he wouldn't be seeing you until this afternoon. Aren't you going to ask me in?"

"Of course, Mrs. Acton!"

I stepped hastily out of the widening pool I stood in. "I'm sorry—I worked late last night and just got up! I thought you were Anne, my next-door neighbor. We both studied late last night, and we borrow books from each other. . . . Will you please make yourself at home while I dress? I won't be a moment."

She nodded and walked gingerly around the damp patch, to stare around my cramped apartment curiously.

"Please sit down, Mrs. Acton. Would you like some coffee? I won't be a moment." She was choosing a place to sit as I dashed for the bedroom.

My face was still red, I noticed in the mirror as I toweled myself dry, standing on the mat beside my still-unmade bed. Then I began to dress hastily.

"I came around for a little chat with you, Samantha." I could still hear her voice saying that. About what? It seemed to me I didn't have to guess. I knew. She didn't want me to marry Paul. She didn't think I was good enough for her son, heir to the Acton wealth and all that. And my hurried appearance to greet her, wrapped in a bath towel, hadn't helped my image any.

Dressing hurriedly in a skirt and sweater, brushing my thick hair into some semblance of order, I could feel myself becoming angrier and angrier. Who did she think she *was* to arrange our lives for us? I loved Paul, and Paul loved me! That had nothing to do with any social order of things. What was she going to try? To buy me off, the way they wrote about in nineteenth-century fiction? Or try to discredit me with Paul? How disappointed she must have been, looking around my apartment from the doorway and not finding Paul, *or preferably some other man in here!*

I took a quick look at my angry face in the mirror and came out fighting.

"What was it you wanted to have your little chat with me about, Mrs. Acton?" I demanded, too angry to conceal the way I felt. "About Paul?"

She had chosen the small sofa to sit on, and to my astonishment, she began to laugh at me. She had a mellow, pleasant laugh that checkmated me abruptly and efficiently.

She patted the cushions beside her, and the laugh became an almost schoolgirlish giggle.

"Come and sit beside me for a moment. The coffee will keep. Why would I want to talk to you about my son? I know him better than you do."

"Then what . . . ?" I puzzled, forced to fight to keep my anger.

"I came here to talk to you about yourself, Samantha." She giggled again. "I'm sorry I came here without warning, but how else could I see you? Paul said the apartment doesn't have a phone. All I could get from him was your address. When you answered the door like that, I knew just how you must feel, seeing me standing there. But it was too late then." She shook her head, studying me. "Sorry about that, Samantha."

"That's all right, Mrs. Acton," I muttered, thrown into confusion by her change of mood.

"I was so *sure* you were Anne. But so long as you didn't mind . . . ?"

"Mind?" she said, giggling outrageously now. "I thought it was *hilarious*! If you could have seen your expression when you recognized *me*!"

It began to seem funny to me too as I thought about it now. I began to giggle too, involuntarily. "Was I as obvious as that, Mrs. Acton?"

"If I'd laughed, you would never have forgiven me," she said. "And just now, when you were so angry with me, you looked as though you were quite sure I detested you and that my only concern was in breaking up your marriage by fair means or foul."

"I don't know what to say, Mrs. Acton!" I muttered, embarrassed.

"I came here because I *want* to like you, Samantha," she told me quietly. "To do that, I need to know much more about you than Paul is likely to tell me. Paul is prejudiced where you're concerned, you know. But as I told him on the phone this morning, I want to know all about a girl I hope can become the daughter I never had."

I stared at her, brought close to tears suddenly as I remembered my own mother. "Mrs. Acton, that's the nicest thing anyone has ever said to me," I said softly.

The ice between us had broken. I found myself talking about my parents as I'd never been able to do before, even to Paul. I told her about the way their marriage had broken up, how they'd separated, divorced, and each married again. I was left in the middle, enrolled at Stanford without money of my own, my mother in New York, my father in Europe. I felt I must graduate. I didn't want to go with either, even if they wanted me, and because of their new partners, neither did.

She was easy to talk to; she said the right things in the right places. I was entranced by a charming new Vanessa Acton whose understanding was smothering my doubts. When I told her how, realizing I had to have a scholarship to go on, I applied for and won one, she expressed sympathy and admiration for what I had achieved alone and unaided.

"You must stay with me at Los Angeles, Samantha," she urged me. "We live on an estate my husband bought in Bel Air. Perhaps at the end of the semester? But we can talk about that at dinner, can't we? I asked Paul if you would both have dinner with me tonight. He said he would if you agreed. I'd love to have you, Samantha."

How could I refuse?

Later, as I walked her downstairs to where a chauffeur waited with a hired black limousine that looked a block long, she flashed me her dazzling smile and kissed me lightly on the cheek.

"You must call me Vanessa, *not* Mrs. Acton, Samantha," she told me with a smile. "I like for the people I love to call me Vanessa. Even Paul calls me that—except when I annoy him, as I did yesterday at the hotel!" Her lovely eyes crinkled at the corners as she studied me. "I believe I was a little jealous! Wasn't that foolish of me?"

I walked slowly back upstairs, still a little dazed, and with the smell of her exotic perfume lingering.

2

The dinner with Paul's mother at the St. Francis was perfect. She was as attentive to me as she was to Paul. It was as though we three had been a family for ages, dining together the way we were. Like the family she said she wanted us to be.

This must have seemed to Paul just the right moment to bring out the ring he'd bought me, and put it on my finger, with Vanessa watching intently. When she had admired it, Vanessa ordered champagne.

My cup of happiness was full as she proposed a pretty toast to us both and we sipped our Dom Perignon.

"Paul," she decided as we sat back, "why don't we have Samantha stay with us at Bel Air for the summer vacation?"

"Why not?" Paul said, grinning at me delightedly.

I smiled at them both affectionately. "I'd like to Vanessa, but I'm afraid that's impossible," I confessed, coming back from dreams to reality, like Cinderella at midnight, as I remembered. "As you know, I'm at Stanford on a scholarship, and I work part time in the library. The scholarship covers only my college tuition. I need to work for living expenses. You see, even if I graduate now, I'll need postgraduate training for another year at least to become a fully trained librarian. I can't afford to stop work this vacation, much as I'd love to."

"I could help you, Samantha," she said seriously, looking deeply into my eyes. "I would like to."

"I couldn't let you do that, Vanessa."

"If Paul graduates, as I'm sure he will—will you still need to work all vacation?"

Sitting beside me, Paul found my hand and squeezed it in approval. "Vanessa, it may be some time before I'm accepted and able to work in my profession. And earn," he said. "We want to wait for that. We have plenty of time. Later, Samantha will work too, and we'll really get ourselves established."

"This is what you both want?" She looked at me, not at Paul.

"I know it's what *I* want, Vanessa," I told her gently.

"We planned it that way," Paul said.

Studying us both impartially, she smiled. "I admire you both," she said. "And I respect your wishes. But remember, if it doesn't work out, if things go wrong, helping you would be my pleasure. Money is no problem. You can open your own office, Paul. In whatever city you fancy."

Paul smiled affectionately. "That isn't the way I want to do it, Vanessa. I know my own limitations. I'm not ready for that yet. I need more experience, and the way to do that is start at the bottom in someone else's office. What I'd like most is to start with some firm of corporate lawyers in San Francisco, so I can be close to Samantha. Once I start work, we can marry. I can commute from here into the city."

Vanessa sighed and looked at her wrist-watch, encrusted with diamonds larger than mine. "I waited till after dinner to tell you, but I'm flying home tonight. I'll have to say good-bye."

"Vanessa," Paul said anxiously, "when will we see you again? Are you coming back to see me get my diploma—if I make it?"

She laughed softly, affectionately. "What a question! And what's this about watching *you* get your diploma? Now I have *two* of you to watch parade in your caps and gowns. And did you say *if*, Paul Acton? There's no way two young people with your kind of determination and the incentive you have could *ever* fail."

We said good-bye to Vanessa in the lounge, and she kissed us both and said she wouldn't wish us luck because she *knew* we'd both pass.

It had been one of the best days of my life, I realized, when back home in the apartment I slid in between the sheets. A mixed day, but a good day. And certainly one day I'd never forget, from the time I opened my door to see Vanessa Acton standing outside, until her son, Paul, kissed me good night outside the apart-

ment and told me for the nth time how much
he loved me.

The last days of the semester dragged wea-
rily to an end. Paul and I were both studying
too hard to see each other. We worked long
hours, and our only contact was when, almost
falling asleep in the library over some textbook
while I waited for customers, I would hear the
phone ring and know it would be Paul. We'd
compare notes, kiss each other long distance,
and go back to our books and our notes until
nature defeated us and we crawled back to our
respective apartments and fell into bed.

Occasionally I saw Vanessa's name mentioned in the social columns, but Paul never
heard from her. He said she was probably too
busy to phone, and she hated writing letters, so
never did. Then, on the last night, when the
phone burred in the library and the girl on the
switchboard beckoned me, a woman's voice answered instead of Paul.

"Could I speak to Samantha Walton,
please?"

There was no mistaking that cultured voice.
"This is Samantha speaking, Vanessa," I said,
delighted. "How are you?"

"Exhausted, darling!" she said. "Never seem
to have a moment. It must be almost the end of
the semester—how do you feel? Confident?"

"I wish I did," I confessed. "I've got the
exam jitters. Doubts. It was harder than I
thought."

"And Paul? I haven't heard from him. I thought he'd phone."

"He seems to be sure he's going to pass. I haven't seen him lately. We've both been too busy. But he phones me. He's very confident."

He always is," she said. "So am I. He'll make it. So will you. Give him my love."

"Of course."

"I'll see you in cap and gown, then. *Both* of you."

"I hope so!"

"Afterward, we'll have dinner again together. I'm looking forward to another chat with you, Samantha."

I remembered that Paul wanted us to celebrate alone together that night, because, as he said, that was *our* grand finale.

But what else could I say except: "I'd like that too, Vanessa."

"I think I've found a way out of our difficulties," she said in her calm voice.

"Oh? In what way, Vanessa?"

But she was gone. The phone clicked as she hung up.

I shrugged. Vanessa, her son said, was always on the go, always too busy to make even a long telephone conversation. Still, it had been good to hear from her again. And Paul could fight it out with her about what we did on the night of our grand finale. Now that his mother and I were friends, I wanted no quarrel with her about anything like that. Let it be Paul's choice, not mine. I was neutral!

My results came through first, and I barely

had courage to open the envelope. But I had passed, with distinction in two subjects, and was tenth in my class. We celebrated that night, Paul and I. He was anxious—I sensed it—but he still thought he'd pass.

He did! *Magna cum laude,* and in second place! An honors pass. After that, the actual presentation seemed in the nature of an anticlimax. The strain caught up with us both, and we offered no resistance at all when, after the procession and the presentations, a smiling and fashionably dressed Vanessa offered to buy us dinner.

We both agreed meekly.

It was quite a night. Other graduates were there too, celebrating as we were, but Paul and Vanessa and I saw only one another. Toward the end, following the champagne, we began to mix. It was while some of Paul's classmates drew him away from us to another table that Vanessa and I had the little chat she'd promised me.

"Now that we're alone, Samantha," she said, leaning toward me conspiratorially, "I would like to tell you about an idea that has occurred to me. I know how tired you must be after all that study and stress. You need a vacation. I mean a real vacation, where you can swim and sunbathe, and relax. You can swim, can't you?"

I smiled. "I can swim, Vanessa, but I told you why I can't accept your invitation to spend the summer with you. I need to work. That's part of our plan to be self-supporting. I want to help Paul, not leave everything to him. The way I feel, the way we both feel, we want our marriage to be a partnership."

"Samantha," she said anxiously, "what I have in mind is a way you can enjoy that kind of vacation and yet at the same time earn as much money as you do in the Stanford library. I think it's a brilliant idea, Samantha! And I know you'd like the work."

I had been studying her calm, guileless face suspiciously.

"No charity, Vanessa?"

"Charity? Who said anything about charity?" She looked hurt.

I explained, not without guilt born of that expression of hurt: "I know how much you want to help us, Vanessa, and how kind you are!"

That seemed to please her, for she smiled. But I was learning that it was hard to tell what thoughts were behind that placid expression on Vanessa's lovely face.

She glanced around, checking on Paul. She found him deep in conversation at a table at the far end of the restaurant. She nodded, satisfied that he couldn't intrude on what she had to say.

"David, my late husband, bought a beach house down on the coast south of Pescadero," she said. "Actually, it's not just an ordinary beach house—it's more like a mansion. He thought it had great potential as an investment in real estate. It also had a fine library built up by the original owner before it came into the hands of the people David bought it from. The original owner collected rare books, a hobby he could afford. He was a wealthy man. David thought the library could be as valuable as the property. He intended to restore the house and the library." She hesitated. "Unfortunately . . . David died a week after the sale went through."

"I'm sorry, Vanessa," I murmured, embarrassed by her distress.

She shook her head. "Paul had just started college. He had his plans, his career. *I* had nothing when David died." Momentarily there was an edge of bitterness in her voice that shocked me; then she smiled. "But that isn't what I want to talk to you about, Samantha. On this day we don't want any morbid thoughts, do we?"

"I know how I would feel if Paul—"

"Don't say that, Samantha!" She glanced across the room at Paul before she looked at me. "I was with David when he bought Finisterre, as the house is called. Since his death, I've never been back to Finnisterre, and Paul has never even seen the place. It's rather inaccessible, a great rambling mansion with its own private beach, far from the congestion and pollution of popular beach resorts. David put in a housekeeper and some staff, and I've kept them there. Paul often asks me why I don't sell the place, but I . . . well, for sentimental reasons I can't do it."

"I think I'd feel the same way."

"Will you spend the summer there, Samantha?" she asked me quietly. "Will you examine, repair, and catalog the library books the way David intended? I'll pay whatever you think the work is worth. I'll buy whatever materials you need, arrange for an assistant to help you. The housekeeper, Mrs. Hacha, has a son who could be very useful. David said he knows every book in the library, and he has attempted to restore some himself. All the rest of the staff will have done is dust the backs of the books on their shelves. You would be protecting an asset that will be Paul's and yours one day. What do you say, Samantha?"

"I . . . don't know, Vanessa. I'd have to talk to Paul."

"You'd be well looked after. You could use the beach whenever you wished. I'm sure Mrs. Hacha and her staff do. The few days David and I spent together there were wonderful. The beach faces east. The sun is on it all day long. It's a wonderful experience having a beach all to yourself, Samantha."

"I can imagine! But . . ."

"You will be doing me a great favor. I mean it. While you are there, I'll spend as much time with you as I can. I think . . . I feel that with you there I can overcome my reluctance to go near Finisterre. And if you are there, can you imagine Paul keeping away? Even if he gets the appointment he wishes in some corporate attorney's office in the city, I guarantee he'll spend his weekends at Finisterre. Especially when he sees the place for himself, and uses the beach."

She studied my face anxiously. "Please, Samantha . . . ?"

"Okay," I said. "If Paul agrees, *I'll do it.*"

She smiled and patted my hand across the table. "Samantha, I'm so grateful, I just don't have words to tell you. How much do they pay you at Stanford? I'll double that, and—"

I laughed. "Really, Vanessa! *No.* I'll accept what I earn at Stanford, but no more. It's just enough." I noticed Paul turning toward us. "I think Paul's coming back!"

"Samantha, I've just thought of something important. You can't go down there until I've checked that Finisterre is fit for you to live in. Anything can happen to a house when you leave paid help to look after it and don't go near the place for years. Let's say nothing about it to Paul at this stage, shall we? Not until I'm sure it's fit to live in? I know how Paul would love to have it so we can get together there at weekends, the three of us. And I know just how disappointed he'd be if I went down there and found it badly neglected—if after telling him about it, we can't do it."

"Well . . ."

"Promise, Samantha? Don't say anything to Paul *yet*?"

I smiled. Paul was coming back, hurrying as he realized how long he'd been away. I smiled at Paul reassuringly.

"Very well, Vanessa," I said. "We'll do it your way."

"Now that I've made up my mind about Finisterre—thank you, Samantha!" she said. "That place will live again, thanks to you. I'll phone you as soon as I've been down there. Right?"

"Right," I said.

Some of the other people came over then, and there were introductions. I noticed the men studying Vanessa, and I could understand why. It seemed impossible that she could be Paul's mother. Paul was twenty-four, and when she was smiling and happy, as she had become since I gave in to her wishes, Vanessa could have passed for an attractive woman in her thirties. Her skin was without a blemish, and I knew lots of women in their twenties who would envy her figure. When you added her poise, sophistication, and self-confidence, you didn't have to ask why she was the center of attention.

Vanessa went rushing back to Los Angeles that night, and we saw her off at the airport. It was great having time on our hands after those days of frenzy. It meant we could see each other every day, without having to hurry back to our roosts to study or to rest for the stresses of next day's classes.

I was off work at the library for a few days while they were doing some vacation-time repairs. And now the offers started to come in from firms wanting Paul to go to work for them.

We read and studied them together over lunch in our favorite Palo Alto coffee shop. Both of us glowed with pride that the letters were from important law firms who wanted not just any graduate, but the best. And because of his results, they had chosen Paul. We argued

interminably, accepting and rejecting the offers.
One was too far away, another not quite in the
top bracket of law firms, a third seemed too in-
definite . . .

We'd read them through and start again.
Paul wanted an offer from San Francisco, I
knew, to be close to me. But so far, nothing exciting had arrived from San Francisco at all.
Paul kept telling me that one must come, unless
the Berkeley graduates were all geniuses this
year. But I was beginning to opt for Los Angeles, from where already he had several invita-
tions to interviews. I would be lonely in Palo
Alto with my postgraduate studies, but after
all, it *was* our whole future we were trying to
plan. And that could depend on the kind of
start Paul got.

It was decided for us, I knew, when I was
called to the phone in the Stanford library and
heard Vanessa's voice, full of triumph and ex-
citement.

"Samantha? I've the most wonderful news!
John Harding, of Harding, Harding, and Chadwick, the corporate attorneys who handle all
David's and my investments and business legal-
ities, called me today. He wants Paul to fly
down to Los Angeles tonight. He's going to offer him a place in the firm commensurate with
the ability he's shown in doing so well in law
school. Isn't it fantastic?"

"Wonderful," I said cautiously, but remembering what Paul wanted most. "Do they have
an office in San Francisco?"

"They're one of the biggest and most impor-

tant legal firms in this country, Samantha," she
said primly. "They have offices *everywhere!*
Washington, Boston, New York, Miami, Mon-
treal, London . . . Paul was most excited
when I told him. Has he phoned you yet? I
told him to."

"Not yet."

"He will. Samantha, I've a confession to
make. I've been working on John Harding all
week, so just haven't had time to drive to Finisterre about the library thing. I'm awfully
sorry."

"That's all right, Vanessa."

"I'm doing something about that right now,
though. Paul's appointment is for tomorrow
morning. I've booked him on the flight to Los
Angeles tonight, and he'll stay at home in Bel
Air. He'll be back for the weekend *with the job*,
I promise you! Meantime, I'll meet you both at
San Francisco airport with Paul's tickets; I'm
booked on the earlier flight to San Francisco. A
car will be waiting to drive me to Finisterre
when Paul's gone. You've been very patient.
Can you be patient till the weekend, then we
can tell Paul our little secret together?"

"Of course, Vanessa."

"I'll see you tonight, then."

She was no sooner off the phone than Paul
called. He said he'd been madly packing. He
sounded as excited about it as Vanessa. But it
was going to be a rush to catch the plane, and
he wanted us to have a few minutes alone together before Vanessa arrived. That meant I
had to rush too, to get Anne Amberg to the li-

brary to stand in for me. I made it with only a few minutes to spare. We sipped coffee in the airport lounge, both of us coming slowly back to earth again after rushing like crazy to be where we were. When Vanessa was about, there was never a dull moment, it seemed to me.

"Are you pleased?" I asked Paul as we sat down.

"They're one of the most important legal firms there is. I couldn't do better, Samantha," he said earnestly.

"Then I'm glad for you, Paul. I asked your mother if they had an office in San Francisco. She said they have offices *everywhere*."

"*Except* San Francisco," he said. "I checked."

"Then we'll be separated for a while?" I asked, not showing the way I felt about that.

"Wouldn't you like that, Samantha?" His gray eyes quizzed me, hiding something.

"I can put up with it. If it's for the common good."

"It is, it will be, we'll make it be!" he said, grinning. "I'll be working at law the way I wanted it, Samantha, if I get the job."

"Vanessa is sure you will."

He frowned. "I see! Then she pulled strings, brought pressure on Harding. She is an important client of Harding, Harding, and Chadwick. You noticed they didn't write to me? They don't have to. The graduates write to Harding, Harding, and Chadwick if they want an appointment for an interview. They take their pick of the applicants. I don't like doing things this way, Samantha."

"I didn't think you would."

"But if I take it, I believe I can prove to Mr. Harding that he made the right choice."

"I'm sure you can!" I saw he liked the way I said that.

"There's the matter of you here and me there, though," he said.

"We'll find a way," I told him with certainty.

He smiled, delighted. "If *you* say so, we will! One hour by plane—that's nothing. Look! We could get married right away, anytime. I'll be earning enough to rent an apartment in Los Angeles, and we could live comfortably on my salary. Or we could each do our own thing, and commute to get together weekends. It depends on what we both want."

"Like togetherness?"

"Exactly," he said. "Or like your graduate studies and my career in law. But if it becomes unbearable apart, I want *you* to make the choice. Okay?"

I said, "It's a pity they don't have an office in San Francisco, isn't it?"

"Yes. Then everything would be perfect."

"Maybe *you* can open one here when you're made junior partner?" I suggested.

He laughed. "Just give me six months, Samantha!" he said, grinning. "I'd better meet her now, her plane's in. Coming?"

We met Vanessa hand-in-hand.

Watching her elegant form coming down the steps, Paul said quietly, "I have to be grateful to her for what she's done. For using her influence on my behalf with Harding. It means two things I like, Samantha. It means we're independent the day I start with Harding. We can marry in a month. *Remember that!* All we have to do is decide which way we go, yours or mine."

"Or *ours*," I reminded him, wondering suddenly if Vanessa too had seen it that way, as a choice between our two careers. "What's the second thing you like, Paul?"

"It means Vanessa has accepted you, completely, as her future daughter-in-law." He smiled. "I told you she never before showed the slightest approval of any girl of mine."

Greeting a smiling Vanessa, I found myself wondering about that too.

3

"I'll see you in three days in the library! Four at the most, Samantha!"

I wakened with Paul's voice calling that to me as he had at the airport when we parted. I had been dreaming of Paul, a pleasant dream that his voice calling had taken away. I wakened resentfully. I yawned and stretched unhappily. Everyone seemed to have deserted me. Ann Amberg had taken the opportunity of Paul's being away to visit an aunt over in Oakland. While *I* had nothing else to do but work, she said. Not that I minded, really. I owed Anne the time. She'd often been my stand-in while I was on unexpected dates with Paul.

It was not just Anne who had deserted me, either. Paul hadn't phoned. I couldn't understand why. I had even walked down to the Palo Alto post office and checked out the Los Angeles directory for the Acton phone number in exclusive Bel Air. There was no V. Acton listed. But that didn't help me any, as another day passed and Paul neglected to call me.

I kept expecting Vanessa to phone the library, but she did not. I was beginning to worry about her too. Surely she couldn't still be at the beach house with the strange name? Finisterre. They called beach houses by all sorts of imaginative names like Shangri-la, or Golden Sands, or even Wait-a-While, but to call a beach house *Finisterre*? Corrupted from the Latin, it couldn't mean much else than "The End of the Earth," could it? Well!

My anxiety and impatience prompted me to walk down to the post office again twice after lunch, as I remembered that I could find the phone number of the office of Harding, Harding and Chadwick. But when I got there and found the number in the Los Angeles directory, I couldn't bring myself to make the call. Paul could be in the middle of some important conference, and I didn't want to endanger his job in any way. I kept assuring myself he'd call me anytime now. Maybe even while I was at the post office. I hurried back home.

I saw the car parked outside the apartment house the moment I turned the corner. It had to be Vanessa's, because there was a chauffeur reading a newspaper behind the wheel. He looked over his newspaper at me as I opened the door to speak to him, a man in his fifties with graying black hair, his cap beside him on the seat.

"Excuse me. Is this Mrs. Acton's car?"

"Yes, miss." He put down his paper quickly and smiled at me. "Are you Miss Walton, apartment seventeen?"

"Yes, I am." I smiled in relief. "Is Vanessa
... Mrs. Acton upstairs?"

"She's in the city on business, miss. She sent
me here with a letter for you. The lady in the
office has it. She said I should wait out here if I
wanted an answer."

"Where can I see Mrs. Acton?"

He shook his head. "I wouldn't know, miss.
But maybe that's in the letter. All I know is, I'm
supposed to drive you to Finisterre, and be
back in San Francisco when the business conference and the dinner Mrs. Acton is attending
ends around ten-thirty tonight. We're driving
home to Bel Air then. Mrs. Acton is a busy
woman."

"She expects me to go to Finisterre? Now?"

"This afternoon, miss. Otherwise, I won't be
in San Francisco at ten-thirty. You are the
young lady who's going to work in the library,
aren't you?"

I frowned. "That wasn't definite." I watched
him register surprise.

"She's been working down there for days, fix-
ing things up for you," he said accusingly.
"And everyone else down there. She's sure
you're going with me, or she wouldn't have sent
me to pick you up."

"There seems to be a misunderstanding," I
said, remembering that I had said I would do it
if Paul agreed. My promise to her had prevent-
ed me from telling Paul anything about it. She
hadn't even released me from that same
promise yet. Had she told Paul, had he agreed?

The chauffeur smiled affectionately. "Mrs.

Acton is an impulsive lady. But very kind. She's good to work for. She's been refurnishing a bedroom for you, supervising all the work herself. She's like that. And Adrian Hacha—that's the housekeeper's son—and I have been carting crates of stuff from the city for your work in the library."

"I'll read the letter. Can you wait?"

"Of course. I asked the lady in the office if I could carry your things downstairs when you pack. She said I could."

I picked up the letter from the apartment superintendent, Mrs. Pettit, and took it upstairs to my room away from her obvious curiosity.

"Are you going away for the summer holidays, Miss Walton?" she asked as she gave it to me. "The man in the car outside seemed to think you are."

"I haven't made up my mind yet, Mrs. Pettit."

"I wouldn't have to think twice in your shoes," she called after me enviously. "Everyone seems able to get away from this place except *me!*"

Upstairs I stopped at Anne's apartment, intending to read my letter there and ask Anne's opinion before I decided. I remembered Anne wasn't there.

In the peace of my own little apartment I perched on the arm of the sofa and opened the envelope.

"Dear Samantha," I read. "So sorry I haven't been able to contact you sooner, but I've been awfully busy, and the phones at Finisterre are hopeless. I arranged for the telephone company to send a technician, but as of this morning he hasn't appeared yet.

"First, a message from Paul! He said he wanted to phone you at night when you're in the library, but that was only possible on one occasion, as he too has been busy nights, and then the girl who answered said you hadn't arrived yet."

I remembered that, smiling. I'd been delayed. Poor Paul, he must be as worried as I'd been! I read on.

"I'm to tell you that he has the job! Then what will probably seem to you the bad news—he has to start work immediately. His first job is to accompany one of the senior executives to attend a court case in Phoenix, Arizona. He will be away at least two weeks, and he was leaving with Mr. Carson on the three-thirty-P.M. flight from LA. I told him to be sure and phone you before the plane left, so no doubt you will learn this from Paul yourself."

I looked at the clock in my bedroom. Three-forty—his plane was gone!

"*Oh no!*" I said aloud. The phone must have been ringing while I was walking back from the post office! Perhaps even while I was talking to the chauffeur downstairs. I turned back to Vanessa's letter, close to tears.

"The beach house is in much better shape now than it was when I came here the night Paul left for LA, despite the fact that I seemed to have been commuting to Bel Air (twice!) since. At least I've refurnished a suite with a

view for you, even though it's only with furniture chosen from other rooms. I think you'll like
it here. I'm going to have to miss seeing you today, as I have to attend a board meeting in San
Francisco this afternoon, followed by a dinner
at night, and must commute back to Bel Air afterward. However, I'll join you at Finisterre as
soon as possible, I promise!

"Now, about your work at Finisterre, Samantha. I have a friend in San Francisco who's a
professor of English at Berkeley and a frantic
bibliophile. I persuaded him to come down
here and advise me what was needed. On his
advice, I've bought supplies, which are ready
for your use. He believes the books should be
valued and insured, as there are many first edi-
tions and some positively antique works. He believes it would be wrong to hurry the work of
restoration, no matter how long it takes. He
told me there's a lot more work than I imagined. He doubts that you can finish it during
the vacation.

"I'm truly grateful that you're doing this for
me, Samantha. I know now how independent
you are, so will not offer you more money than
you ask. But I am determined to make it up
to you, perhaps as a wedding present. Love,
Vanessa."

She had added a postscript.

"Make sure you bring *all* your clothes and
things. Finisterre is isolated. On second
thought, why don't you *give up* that silly little
cramped apartment? That way, you would save
the rent. You have a house and servants here

completely at your service. And who knows, Samantha? With Paul's prospects so bright, you may decide to marry as soon as you are finished with the work here. You could, you know. And then you would be moving to Los Angeles to live where Paul's work is. Why not, Samantha?"

Why not? I thought. *Why not?*

Without making any conscious decision, I began to pack hurriedly. Clothes first, then my books, the few personal things I'd bought over the years to brighten the apartment. Not that I had so much to pack. I brought the first packed suitcase downstairs to the office, and Mrs. Pettit sent the chauffeur up for the rest. But I couldn't bring myself to give up the apartment the way Vanessa suggested. Not until I'd talked to Paul. We had our plan, Paul and I, and my staying another year at Stanford was part of that.

While the chauffeur put my luggage in the trunk of the car, I made a hasty call to Mr. French, the Stanford librarian. With Anne away, it meant he had to find someone at short notice to take my place. Mr. French was most understanding about it as I explained my predicament. He said it was okay, though he was sorry he was losing me over the vacation period, when most of the students went home. He even asked me to be sure to come back when the new semester started, as he liked my work. I thought maybe the fact that I was going to work in Vanessa's library might have helped. The Actons had been loyal benefactors of Stanford for generations.

The chauffeur drove up to the drugstore to pick me up, to the interest of the clerk behind the counter. I chose to ride beside the chauffeur. I would have needed a telephone to talk to him from the back seat, and I was still curious about what was happening. I noticed that Mrs. Pettit was watching curiously as I got in.

He told me his name was Ed Hart, and he and his family of two sons and a daughter all lived and worked at the Acton place in Bel Air. When he described it to me as we drove, he made it sound like one of the mansions of the film stars. He said he'd hardly seen Paul since he came home. Paul was in the city each day, and he had been dining nights with executives of Harding, Harding and Chadwick.

I had a jealous twinge when he mentioned that Paul and John Harding's daughter, Joanna, had known each other all their lives, so Paul was always welcome at the Harding home. He'd been driving Paul there to dinner, and once, he added with a sidelong glance, he drove the Hardings, Joanna, and Paul to the Coconut Grove because Paul was taking the family to dinner.

That held me silent and resentful all the way to the underpass where we crossed under the Skyline Boulevard at Monte Bello Ridge. After that the mountain scenery held me quite all the way to Pescadero. We turned south at the Coast Highway, following the highway to where Ed slowed at a roadside store and turned off where a battered signpost proclaimed: "Finisterre Point, 2 M."

The mountains had become a herringbone of ridges sloping down to the sea. We followed a gravel road winding through pine forest with no houses in sight. Once, some animal vanished into tangled brush, seen only as a patch of shiny black hair that Ed said laconically he thought might be a bear.

"I've often seen them on this road, since Mr. Acton bought Finisterre," he remarked. "One day, I swear I saw a timber wolf, but Mrs. Acton said it had to be a dog, probably a German shepherd gone wild. She said timber wolves are long gone. All the same, I wouldn't walk this road for a bet."

"Finisterre must be a very isolated place," I muttered. "But there are neighbors, no doubt, and shops someplace?"

"There's just Finisterre," he said, grinning. "The shop back on the Coast Highway is both the nearest shop *and* the nearest neighbor. Mrs. Hacha does most of the shopping in Pescadero, sixteen miles back. They have a pickup truck at the house, but no car unless Mrs. Acton and I are there."

I frowned, considering that. "How do the people who work there get transport home, when they're not working?"

"The pickup drops them at the highway store. Buses go through, both ways. But as I said, I wouldn't recommend that *anyone* walk there."

"It's a wonder people work there," I muttered, staring at the trees pressing in on either side. Beneath and between the spreading branches, the sunlight filtering down gave things a yellowish-green, ghostly look. I shivered for some reason I couldn't understand. I was realizing suddenly that I wasn't sure I wanted to work here, either.

"Work isn't plentiful in these parts, Miss Walton," he said. "They can't pick and choose. And Mrs. Acton is good to work for, as I said. I don't think Mrs. Hacha or her son would want to live anywhere else. Mrs. Hacha knew Mrs. Acton before the Actons bought Finisterre. It wouldn't surprise me if Mrs. Hacha was responsible for Mr. Acton becoming interested in it in the first place."

"Are there other servants?"

"Two maids at present, and an old Mexican I call Pancho, who potters around the garden. One of the maids comes from Pescadero. The other girl's from San Francisco. They come and go. But with the family not in residence, they don't have a lot to do. The food's good, and there's a beach lots of people would give Fort Knox to have in front of their house."

"What's it like? The house, I mean."

"Incredible. You'll see it for yourself as we come over the next ridge."

I was aware of a sense of space ahead as the car climbed smoothly. The late afternoon had passed as we drove, and the light was failing beneath the trees. Beyond the ridge, as we reached the crest, I saw that the trees thinned away to bare, open ground.

"Finisterre!" Ed Hart declared with an unexpected sense of the dramatic.

It was lighter beyond the trees about us, and the road bent down to cliffs at the edge of the sea. And what a sea! The house was there, as he said, directly below and in front of us, an incredible Gothic mansion, complete with cathedrallike spires and towers and all the curlicues and slender piles and buttresses of the Gothic style thrusting up above a high stone wall.

But what astonished me, what held me silent and staring, was the coloring of this lonely house on a cliff with the backdrop of sea behind it. For it was as though the great house was etched in black ink against a sea of milky white in unbelievable contrast.

"Goddamn fog!" Ed Hart muttered disgustedly. "And I have to drive back to San Francisco *tonight*!"

"*That's fog?*" I muttered incredulously. Behind the house, the sea was a perfectly flat expanse of white, not just opaque, but impenetrable, reaching from what I judged must be just below the clifftops out to the far horizon.

"I've seen it looking like that, like a sea of milk, quite often," he said. "Not bad to look at like this, but when night comes, it creeps up out of the sea. In a couple of hours' time, you wouldn't see your nose in front of your face in these woods. I meant to have dinner at Finisterre, like I said—the food's good. But not now. Soon as I carry in your things, Miss Walton, I'm pushing off. I'll have it all the way. I'd bet on it."

"I've never seen fog as thick or as white as that!"

"You'll see it again," he said, glancing at me as we rolled out of the woods and swooped down upon the great iron gates that were the only break I could see in the stone walls surrounding the house.

"Just don't ever stay out in it, either on the beach or up in the woods," he said grimly. "Or, if you do get caught, stay fast wherever you are. Don't try to find your way home through it."

I shivered. "I'm not likely to *go out* in that!"

As I watched, the house lights began to come on in the lower rooms, lights that disappeared as we rolled down the hill and the high stone wall hid them, except for one bright, welcoming light above the gates. Approaching, Ed Hart loosed a blast on the car horn that brought someone in white overalls hurrying from a cottage adjoining the gates to open them. He stared at me curiously as we drove through, a brown-skinned man with lank black hair and brown eyes that shone in the light above the gates.

"Is that Pancho?"

Ed nodded. "The gates are kept locked. Mrs. Hacha's orders."

"I don't blame her. This place is really isolated, and all that woods between here and the highway."

"Well, it's safe enough with the gates locked," Ed said as we drove along a winding drive toward a house that seemed to be growing more gigantic as we approached it. "Those walls are too high to climb, there's glass embedded in concrete on the top, and no trees close enough to help anyone climb over."

He slowed and stopped as we swung around a bend in the drive, and I saw Finisterre at close range for the first time. Steps led up to a massive door that could have belonged to a medieval cathedral.

I stared back in failing light across the neglected grounds through which we had just driven. Only part of the lawns were mowed, and there had been little attempt at gardening for a long time. Shrubs were tall and scraggy; flowerbeds grew weeds taller than the roses fighting for life.

"I'll carry your bags up, Miss Walton. If you go up and ring, one of the maids will come. Mostly they're at the back of the house, so keep your fingers on the bell, if you don't mind. The fog's rising."

He was right about that, I saw as I glanced back toward the section of wall that hid the sea. White veils of fog were already spilling over the wall. I climbed the steps, pressed the bell button, and waiting, heard approaching feet before I released the button and the distant ringing stopped.

"Miss Walton?"

"Yes." The woman who had opened the door to me was in her early forties, a tall, flat-chested woman, with her black hair cut in a severe and mannish style. She had eyes so dark they appeared black. Her clothes matched her eyes, an unattractive black jersey two-piece dress. Those obsidian eyes in an expressionless face, with a thin mouth, studied me disconcertingly.

"We were told to expect you," she said. "I'm Catherine Hacha, Mrs. Acton's housekeeper, and this is my son, Adrian. Adrian, carry Miss Walton's bags up to her room." She glanced back briefly, and I saw the young man standing behind her for the first time as she turned.

"Yes, Mother." He passed me without looking at me; he had the same coloring as his mother, black hair and brown eyes, a suntan that recommended the beach Vanessa had boasted about.

"If you'll follow me, Miss Walton, I'll take you to your room. No doubt you'll want to freshen up before dinner. I'll send a maid up to help you unpack."

"I can manage, thank you, Mrs. Hacha," I said. "No doubt the maid has other things to do."

"Mrs. Acton had to go to San Francisco on urgent business. She said to apologize to you for not being here to greet you. She asked me, in her absence, to make you as comfortable as possible during your stay. The maid will help me do that, as Mrs. Acton wishes. This way please?"

I followed her, feeling politely snubbed. She reminded me of Vanessa the first time I had met her. But Vanessa had thawed toward me, so perhaps this woman would change too.

The passage was wide, and had a high ceiling. Ahead, a chandelier lit a wide staircase. Open doors we passed disclosed vast rooms full of antique furnishings. In one room the furniture was swathed in white sheets, like the ghosts of some dim past that only this house knew about.

Behind us, as we climbed the wide stairway, I heard her son following with my possessions, hurrying to catch up. She climbed quickly, like a man. A strong, still-youthful woman in some ways, I decided, looking for the best in her. And she certainly looked physically fit.

"Mrs. Acton herself chose the rooms you will use, Miss Walton," she said. Her breath was as untroubled as a child's. I noticed, despite a climb that I realized had me breathing hard.

"Yes, I know. She sent me a note by the chauffeur. It was very kind . . . of her." I qualified my previous thought about Catherine Hacha. She did not merely seem physically fit—she was trained like an athlete.

"Vanessa Acton is a fine woman."

"Yes. I think so."

"We have a fine beach here. I swim there a lot. So does my son, Adrian. Do you swim, Miss Walton?"

"Yes."

"Are you a good swimmer?"

What were her standards for good swimming? I wondered. She looked as though she could have been an Olympian. It wasn't wise to boast to someone who looked as fit as she did. After all, the best I'd ever done was win the fifteen-hundred-meters event and the four-hundred for women at college. I had to give up and stop training after last summer because I realized my studies were more important to me. And besides, I'd met Paul.

"Very ordinary," I said.

"Well, no matter." She was studying me obliquely. "Our beach is safe. The sunshine alone makes it a great place to relax."

"I noticed your suntan."

"You can have one, quite easily. We turn here. Your rooms face the sea. She wanted you to have a room on this side of the house. She stayed in here last night. The first night she has spent here since Mr. Acton bought Finisterre. This is your bedroom. . . ."

She was holding the door open for me halfway down the passage from the third-floor landing. Looking around eagerly, I smiled, pleased. The bedroom made a delightful contrast to those rooms I'd glimpsed on my way here, despite its high ceiling and great size. The old-fashioned bed of gleaming redwood shone from polish and care. Everything in the room was spotless, from the obviously new draperies at the window to the bedcovers.

An old-fashioned wardrobe matched the bed, the bedside table, and two huge and comfortable deep chairs.

"Do you like it?"

"Oh, yes, Mrs. Hacha! For the past three years I've been living in a tiny apartment. This is fabulous."

"You have a bathroom over here. The door on the other side of the room opens into a study. Mrs. Acton thought you might need it for your work. I think you'll find that everything you need is here. If not, tell the maid when she comes, and I will attend to it."

"Thank you, Mrs. Hacha, but I'm sure this will be perfect."

My shoes sank in thick new carpet as I crossed the room dutifully to peep into the bathroom and cross to examine the study, while a heavily burdened Adrian Hacha came in with my luggage, and Ed Hart followed with the rest of my gear.

The bathroom had plumbing that was twenties vintage rather than seventies, but it had been recently retiled and was as spotless as the bedroom. The study had the same old-fashioned furnishings, including a huge rolltop desk that could have been the status symbol of some millionaire tycoon at the turn of the century.

"Dinner at seven-thirty, Miss Walton," Mrs. Hacha reminded me. "Please be punctual."

"Of course."

"Hart, since you're not staying for dinner, come to my office. I've a message for Mrs. Acton." She stood poised at the door waiting for him.

I looked around the study. Everything I might need to work in here at night, researching for the library catalog, seemed to be ready for me. Coming back into the bedroom, I walked to the window and drew back the draperies.

Darkness had come while I inspected my rooms, and the fog had crept across the lawns to the house, reaching above the ground-floor windows. All I could see was the glimmer of light from the windows down there and the lamp above the iron gates at the entrance to Finisterre.

"In the morning you will find the view from your windows most impressive, Miss Walton."

Mrs. Hacha was turning, with the chauffeur following. He smiled at me and said good night.

I agreed with the housekeeper about the view. Even in the gloom outside I had the sense of vast space below and beyond the walls of Finisterre, where fog hid the ocean. The sound of the sea against cliffs came up to me through the fog, muted by it, so that it was as though the sea breathed heavily, patiently, waiting. . . .

I shivered and began to turn away, and noticed the cold dampness of the windowsill as my hand touched it. I looked down, puzzled.

Cement, fresh cement, barely dry?

From the door Adrian Hacha's voice, showing eagerness to please me, explained ingenuously. "She had the bars in here taken out especially for you, Miss Walton!"

"Bars?" I turned quickly to stare at him. "Did you say bars?"

"*Adrian!*" his mother's voice called sternly from the passage. He turned at once and followed her silently before I could question him.

Bars? Perhaps I'd misunderstood. I thought of the study windows and went back in to take a look. In there the windowsill was as freshly cemented. It was the same above the window and on either side. Even the small bathroom window had been done in the same way.

While I wondered about that, someone knocked lightly on my door, and a blond girl in a maid's uniform came in carrying a tray with a cup of steaming, fragrant coffee and a cookie.

"Mrs. Hacha said I was to help you unpack, miss." She smiled. "I'm Sara Sheridan. I thought some coffee might help after your drive."

"Thank you, Sara," I said. "And you are so right. Coming to Finisterre for the first time is quite an experience. Coffee is exactly what I need."

"I'll put it on your table in the study."

"I'll wash my hands. There's wet cement around the windows, and I touched it. Adrian Hacha said Mrs. Acton had some bars taken away?"

She nodded, as though that was the most natural thing. "Yes, she did. All the other rooms still have them, but they don't bother anyone. At least, if you lock your door at night downstairs, you know nobody outside can get in."

"You mean that was the purpose of the bars? To keep intruders out?"

She frowned and glanced at the door and lowered her voice. "You don't know about Finisterre? I was sure you would, you being Mrs. Acton's future daughter-in-law. Finisterre was a sanatorium before Mr. Acton bought it. The bars were to keep the patients *in*, not to keep people *out*. Not then."

I stared at her, startled. "What sort of a sanatorium, Sara?"

"Well . . ." She hesitated, and glanced at the open door again uneasily. "Maybe I wasn't supposed to tell you. But nobody said not to. Finisterre was a mental hospital, Miss Walton. It was a place where they put incurable mentally ill patients from wealthy families. They lived and died here. There's a cemetery in the grounds where they were buried."

"A mental hospital?" I stared at her incredulously, and felt myself shiver.

She nodded. "Scary, isn't it? I know it frightens me nights, when I wake in the dark and think about it, when maybe in the next room someone is talking in their sleep. My room is next to Mrs. Acton's suite, and she has bad dreams."

I shook my head. "I suppose we can't blame the house for that," I said. "And if the rest of you can work here and get used to the idea of what Finisterre was once, so can I."

She smiled and studied my face with approval as I sat down to the coffee. "I'll tell you one thing, Miss Walton," she said. "It's good to have someone to wait on in this place, someone *other* than Mrs. Hacha and Adrian, that is. I don't like Adrian. He's a creep. Though the other girl who works here, Jane Buchan, likes him well enough. But it's all right for the Hachas! Adrian was *born* here. His mother was head nurse in the sanatorium in those days. When the Actons bought Finisterre, she and

Adrian stayed on. Would you like me to run your bath?"

She stayed and chattered on, a girl obviously starved for conversation in this great lonely house that had once held the mentally ill. The tortured and the damned of our modern society, as someone described their plight.

I only half-listened as she talked, thinking about this thing.

I was still thinking about it when, hours later, with a dinner that I'd eaten in solitary state in a dining room that could have fed a regiment, I came back to my lonely, isolated rooms two floors above the others and crept into my bed.

4

It had been late last night before I slept. Thinking about the poor people incarcerated for long years behind bars in this great house, perhaps in these very rooms in which I lay sleepless, it was impossible to fall asleep. I had left my windows open earlier, and the cold dampness of fog crept into the room. I had only to close the window, I knew, but my cowardice wouldn't let me get out of bed to do it.

The house, like any old building, was full of small, scary sounds that nudged my nervousness each time I almost dozed. Sounds I imagined my predecessors could have made, like the sighs of the lonely, the unintelligible mutterings of the sick, the faint groans of the hopeless, the pad of sly footsteps, the creak of a board . . .

I seemed barely to have dozed when the maid coming in with early-morning coffee wakened me in such fright that I almost leaped out of bed. The maid, I saw as I returned to earth, was a different girl this morning, a pert and pretty brunette with large but rather insipid

gray eyes, who repressed a giggle at the way
I'd reacted to her unexpected entrance. Her
breasts thrust out the prim maid's uniform, revealing a gold cross on a thin chain at the cleft.

"Good morning, miss. Did I frighten you? I
knocked, but you didn't seem to hear. Mrs.
Hacha said I should bring your coffee up early,
as Mrs. Acton wants you to start work in the library this morning."

"It's perfectly all right. It was just that I
didn't sleep very well last night. I suppose it
was the strange bed."

She smiled. "Nobody sleeps well on their first
night in Finisterre. I know *I* didn't! But you get
used to it. Would you like your coffee in bed?
You might as well." She set it up for me on the
night table.

"Thank you . . . ?" I studied her inquiringly.

"Jane, miss. I'm Jane Buchan." She moved
the table. "There, how's that? Would you like
me to draw the curtains?"

"Has the fog gone? I never saw fog like we
had last night before!"

"Quite gone. See for yourself." As she parted
the drapes to show me, bright sunlight
streamed into my bedroom from a cloudless
sky, almost blinding me. "Great day for a
swim," she added, staring out. "The view from
this window is fantastic. You get the feeling
you can see halfway to Hawaii! I never tire of
looking at it."

"This I have to see!"

I pulled my robe on over my nightgown and

carried my coffee over to join her at the window. Last night I hadn't been able to see anything for fog, but it was different this morning. The Pacific was at its incredible best, blue beneath a sunny sky.

The beach lay directly in front of my window. Completely private, it bordered an inlet enclosed by high cliffs on either side. From my third-floor window I could see a path and steep steps descending to the back of the idyllic stretch of sand that looked clean and untouched. Rocks showed darkly beneath the water at the foot of the cliffs, but from the beach the sea sloped gently out toward deep water where the small breakers started that fell frothing upon the sand.

"Looks great down there, doesn't it?" the maid said. "A couple of days ago, Mrs. Acton came here for the first time since I've been here. That's when we learned you were coming, miss. She came back and stayed overnight. Another first. That was the day before yesterday. Maybe this place will start to live again now. Did you find the present she left for you?"

"Present? No?"

"It's in the top drawer of the wardrobe. She asked me to make sure you found it this morning. There's a note with it. I'll get it while you finish your coffee." Over her shoulder she added, "I know what it is, because she asked me what color I'd like, since I have coloring like yours. . . . But she wasn't quite right about that. My eyes are just ordinary old gray.

I've never seen eyes as close to violet as yours are."

"You have very nice eyes."

"Not like yours, miss." She came back with a gift-wrapped package and an envelope. "Would you like more coffee?"

"No, thanks."

"Then I'll let you try on your present while I help with the breakfast. Mrs. Hacha said to tell you breakfast is at eight-thirty and—"

"Please be punctual?" I smiled.

She giggled. "That's our Mrs. Hacha," she said.

When she had gone, I perched on the edge of my bed and opened the package and the note. Vanessa had left me a fashionable and very brief red bikini and a note of welcome.

In her note she had written: "By now from your window you will have seen the beach I described to you. Enjoy it while the sun shines, Samantha. As I mean to do when, by being at Finisterre with you, I overcome those memories of David that make me so reluctant to return there.

"The bikini is just in case you neglected to bring one. Red should go well with your black hair and those unusual violet eyes. I'm sure Paul will like it! I'll phone you when I hear from him. Love, Vanessa."

I put the note and the bikini away and began to prepare for my first day at Finisterre. I felt better about that this morning. Sunlight improved Finisterre. I went in almost contentedly for my shower.

I tried not to think about Vanessa's promise to phone me when she heard from Paul. I wondered if she had written the note before the one the chauffeur delivered to me? In that note she had informed me that Paul was on his way to Phoenix, Arizona, for a court case that Harding, Harding and Chadwick expected to last at least two weeks.

I didn't want to think about *that*, because it would be the longest Paul and I had been apart since we fell in love. I supposed glumly, as I ran the shower and adjusted it for warmth, that I was going to have to get used to separations like this when I became Paul's wife and he practiced his profession.

The blond maid was waiting in the dining room when I came down to breakfast. She smiled at me and brought fruit juice and cereal from her tray.

"Were you comfortable in your rooms last night, Miss Walton?"

"Yes, thank you, Sara." I glanced at my solitary place set for breakfast at a huge table covered with a spotless white tablecloth, and confessed, "More comfortable than I am being waited on in here alone. I'd prefer to eat in the staff dining room off the kitchen, where Jane told me this morning the rest of you have your meals."

Sara Sheridan looked shocked. "Mrs. Hacha would never allow that, Miss Walton! You're not *staff*, you're practically one of the Acton family! And no doubt she has orders about you from Mrs. Acton herself."

I had been contemplating a confrontation with Mrs. Hacha about that ever since I first came in the door and saw what looked like a boardroom table with one lonely setting. I changed my mind disgustedly. Sara Sheridan must know more about that sort of protocol than I did.

"I feel I'm imposing on you, making too much work," I explained. "I mean, for the size of Finisterre, you must all have much more to do than wait on me."

"But that's what we're here for, Miss Walton!" she protested. She glanced toward the kitchen. "We like it this way. Honestly!"

"Well, okay! If that's the way everyone wants it."

"It is, Miss Walton. If it's just that you're not used to breakfasting alone and you're lonely, whichever one of us in in here serving will talk to you all you want."

"Okay," I said as she brought me cold milk for the cereal. "Tell me about yourself, Sara. Where are you from?"

She began to chatter obligingly. She was from Pescadero, the town on the Coast Highway we'd passed through yesterday, she told me. Her father was a police lieutenant, and she was engaged to a boy from her hometown who was studying architecture in Fresno. The breakfast passed pleasantly enough with someone my own age to talk to.

Mrs. Hacha came in while I sipped my

coffee, and silenced her with a glance, but it didn't matter then. The housekeeper had come in to tell me that Adrian had opened the library and Mrs. Acton had instructed him to help me in my work. I decided this was her way of reminding me that I was here to work, not to waste the time of her help.

"Has Adrian had any library experience, Mrs. Hacha?" I asked with the same cold politeness she had used on me.

"Professor Carter, Mrs. Acton's friend, said that if Adrian hadn't repaired some of the books, they would have completely lost their value," she told me stiffly. "Adrian has always been very good with his hands. I . . . Mrs. Acton believes that he can be very useful to you, Miss Walton! *If* you can tell him what should be done, she is sure Adrian can do it."

I was tempted to retort, but decided to leave it at that while I thought I was slightly ahead. I had noticed her slip when she almost said she and not Vanessa believed Adrian could be useful to me. I was beginning to wonder who was really mistress of Finisterre, Vanessa or her housekeeper? She turned her back on me and stalked out before I remembered I hadn't asked her where the library was.

Sara told me it was on the second floor. She said the books had been stored in a damp cellar while Finisterre was a mental hospital, but Mr. Acton had had them put back upstairs in the original library, which had been in use as the suite of the superintendent of the sanatorium, a Dr. Kurusu. I expected a library to be downstairs, as one of the principal rooms of the house, but she said she'd heard that the person who collected the books believed the air and light were better upstairs.

And no doubt, I thought, *he* should know. I was beginning to like Sara Sheridan.

Adrian was eagerly waiting at the library door. He had unpacked the filing cabinets for the catalog and the materials the professor had suggested Vanessa buy for me.

"I thought you'd want to see what she bought for you," he said happily, standing up to his ankles in straw and dismembered packing cases.

He looked so like a friendly puppy eager to please that I had to suppress a giggle. "I think we should start by putting all the supplies on the table and clearing away the packing material don't you? We can put the filing cabinets in the corner until we decide where we can use them most efficiently. After that, we'll decide how we can best work at the cataloging."

"I'll do it, Miss Walton!" he said. "You don't need to lift things. Or repair things, or carry heavy books. *I* can do that!"

I couldn't resist his eagerness. I smiled involuntarily. Adrian didn't have to be like his mother. I said, "If you're going to help me in here, Adrian, we'll work together at things like this. That way, we'll get the work done. If there are rare and valuable books here, *we* won't be repairing them—they'll be sent to experts if Mrs.

Acton approves. The same with their valuation."

"Then I can help you with the cataloging?"

"Of course. I want to leave with this room organized so a reader can be given or find any book he or she wants without waste of time. And the work in here won't end when I leave Finisterre, so you may as well learn what you can about cataloging by working with me. That way, you can be the librarian when I'm gone."

"Where will you keep this stuff, Miss Walton?" he asked as we put the glues and brushes, the leather and binding materials on the huge table in the center of the room. "I could get a cupboard from the storeroom. Pancho would help me carry it upstairs."

"Do you have one that matches the color of the table and the wall panels and shelves?"

"I'll find one!"

The cupboard he found was perfect. The morning passed quickly as we positioned the cupboard, the filing cabinets, and the typewriter. Halfway through the morning Mrs. Hacha ushered in Jane Buchan, the brunette maid, who was pushing a trolly with our morning coffee. We took a break, reluctantly, for we both were absorbed in our planning of the necessary ground work still to be done before we would really get started on the cataloging.

Every time I glanced at the shelves of books that lined the big room that could well have served the needs of a community of readers rather than a collector, I wanted to drop everything and start taking books from the shelves.

And Adrian, who seemed to really know, as Vanessa had said, every rare book on the shelves, was as eager to show them to me.

His mother was curt and quite horrible to poor Adrian. She seemed suspicious of his working with me, yet did not attempt to take him away, to find him some other chore, as she could have done easily enough. Jane Buchan was just as objectionable, pouting and giving him black looks because he was working with me. It was as though the two women in his life were ganging up on Adrian, determined to give him a bad time because of me.

I began to feel sorry for Adrian. He seemed a shy and rather timid young man, dominated by his strong-willed mother, who ruled everyone at Finisterre with ruthless determination. She would have liked to treat me in the same way, I was sure. But my relationship with Paul frustrated that.

Adrian's weakness of character aroused sympathy in me that I didn't try to hide. I was as nice as I could be to him as Mrs. Hacha inspected what we had done, and the maid waited angrily for us to finish our coffee. Adrian responded with an eagerness, a doglike devotion, that I began to find embarrassing. I was glad when the two women left us alone again and I could begin to cool Adrian's response.

It was the same when the maid came back upstairs to call us for lunch. It was Jane who waited on me at table, and her jealousy and suspicion showed plainly enough. It was not, I decided, that Jane was in love with poor

Adrian, but because Adrian was the only available male living in the great house.

In the afternoon I began to make a cursory inspection of books taken at random from the shelves. Not that there was any method in their stacking. They had been thrust into the shelves as they were brought up from whatever cellar had held them, without even any attempt at shelving them in alphabetical order.

I worked in my own study that first night. I had decided to use the Dewey decimal classification method in cataloging the collection. That meant that a prefix "subject number" would be given to each book, and they would stand on the shelves in numerical order, with books on the same subject having the same subject number. Rare books, I decided to keep in a separate section so that they could be more easily watched for deterioration. I would use letters for subject prefix symbols on the rare books, then number them.

I went to bed so tired that not even the night noises of Finisterre disturbed me.

I was pleased to see Sara Sheridan's more pleasant face presiding over my breakfast. Last night Jane Buchan had been as disagreeable as she could be without any direct confrontation with me.

After Mrs. Hacha had inspected the dining room briefly and gone back to her own meal, breakfast became quite pleasant with Sara to talk to. Instinctively, we spoke in low voices, though what we said seemed innocent enough to me. Such things as lowered voices, I was discovering, could easily become habit in Finisterre.

Sara had received a letter from her boyfriend in Fresno. She said he was coming home to Pescadero for the weekend, which she wanted to spend at home, but Mrs. Hacha hadn't agreed to let her have the time off yet. She said Mrs. Hacha favored Jane Buchan when it came to weekends off. If Jane was away from Finisterre on weekends, a time when Adrian was more or less free, it was easier for Mrs. Hacha to keep an eye on her son.

Sara remarked that Mrs. Hacha kept poor Adrian too busy on weekdays to even watch Jane sunbathing down on the beach, as she did sometimes at lunchtime.

"Not that they don't get together," Sara told me, with a cautious glance toward the kitchen. "Adrian is like his mother, a very good swimmer. And he has taught Jane until she is almost as good. She even skin-dives with him, using a snorkel and mask. Sometimes I hear him tap on Jane's door in the night, and she gets up and goes down to the beach with him. You wouldn't swim in that spooky place at night in a fit! But *they* do. Mrs. Hacha would murder Adrian if she knew. She's the most suspicious woman."

"I noticed that." I smiled. "It's a wonder she doesn't see the wet towels and swimsuits. She wouldn't miss anything like that, I'd say."

Sara glanced at the door warily. "They don't take any."

"There's someplace down there where they keep them?"

"I mean they don't *use* any. They swim in the nude. Jane told me so once when I let her know I heard Adrian waking her. She says on summer nights when there's no fog, it's great. The water is quite warm, and you feel free and swim better without a bikini. They make love down there afterward. Adrian wants to marry her, she says. But she stalls when he asks her. I don't blame her. Could you imagine spending the rest of your life in Finisterre married to poor Adrian, with Mrs. Hacha for your mother-in-law?"

"*No way!*" I smiled.

"Me neither! What I think will happen is that Jane will just take off one weekend and forget to come back. And soon, I'd say. She's getting restless. I've seen a lot of girls come and go here. I know the signs!"

Privately, I hoped Sara was wrong, as I finished my breakfast and got up. It had occurred to me that Adrian might make *me* the object of his obsession if Jane went. I wanted no part of that.

I studied Adrian in a different light as we worked together this morning. Not that I discovered anything about him that I hadn't noticed before. Previously I'd thought of Adrian as a rather simple young man mooning after Jane but not getting anywhere with her. The thought of Adrian as Jane's secret lover, swimming nude with her from the beach beneath my window late at night, was another thing.

He seemed as naive as ever, so that it was difficult to imagine Jane Buchan being attracted

to him. It had to be the other way around. Jane
was an attractive girl from any male viewpoint,
I admitted. She was pretty in a sullen way, she
had the kind of figure men seemed to like, and
as I'd noticed before, her suntan was out of this
world.

Poor Adrian could arouse my sympathy, but
I couldn't imagine myself falling for him, even
if I wasn't in love with Paul. Adrian was the
thin, wiry type. Unlike his mother, he had a
weak face. A face that seemed to me to match
his character.

I began to realize he had noticed my unusual
interest in him this morning, and was beginning to return it. It took effort to adjust, to
concentrate on my work again, to forget the impression Sara had given me of Adrian the mas-
terful, rather than Adrian the meek.

After all, things and people were seldom
what they seemed.

I found myself studying Jane Buchan in the
same way when halfway through the morning
she came into the library with the morning
coffee. She was one of those busty girls with
rounded hips and heavy but quite shapely legs.
Women, I knew, would think her overweight.
But men thought differently, and it wasn't
women that interested Jane. In my preoccupa-
tion with other things, I hadn't noticed there
was only one cup of coffee on her tray, but
Adrian had.

"Hey!" he puzzled anxiously. "Where's my
coffee, Jane?"

She gave me an oddly triumphant glance, I

thought, as she said, "Your mother says you're to have coffee downstairs with *us*. She wants you to drive the pickup into Pescadero to bring back some groceries she needs."

"But I'm helping Samantha . . . Miss Walton," he said in dismay.

"You *were*, Adrian," she said with an openly vindictive smile at his slip.

"Pancho can take the pickup to town!" he protested angrily. "Why *me*, when we've all this work up here?"

"Hadn't you better ask your mother that? And she said she wants you down there *at once*, so you'd better hurry. She was pouring your coffee as I left, and you know how she is about you letting things get cold and spoil."

Momentarily he appeared about to rebel; then he shrugged. "I'm sorry, Miss Walton!"

I gave him a reassuring smile. "That's all right, Adrian. I can manage here until you get back." I took my coffee from Jane Buchan.

"I'll be back soon after lunch," Adrian promised.

"Don't count on that, Miss Walton," Jane interrupted. "His mother has quite a lot for Adrian to do in town today."

She watched him leave, frowning, before she looked back at me. The smile she flashed at me was so bright it made me suspicious.

I said, "Adrian is becoming so interested in my work that he doesn't like to stop."

"In your *work*?" She stressed the word, but slightly, in a way that went with that artificial smile. "Oh, yes! I've noticed how interested

Adrian is, each time I bring up your coffee, Miss Walton. Would you like more natural light in here? It's a terrific day outside!"

She was giving me more light at once, unasked, drawing back the draperies from the windows. More sunlight than I could use flooded in.

"Thank you."

She stared down. "Look at that blue sea! Isn't it fantastic down there this morning?"

"I haven't noticed."

She giggled. "It's like a painting I saw once of a beach in Tahiti. Only the palm trees and hula girls missing. What do you think of our beach, Miss Walton? And the water—isn't it warm? No big breakers to hurt anyone either, are there?" She turned back to me, smiling. "You have been down for a swim?"

"I'm afraid not, Jane. No time, so far."

She stared at me disbelievingly. "D'you mean to say you haven't tried out your present yet?"

I *had* forgotton the red bikini, I realized guiltily. "Present?" I asked, stalling.

She shook her head at me. "The red bikini Mrs. Acton gave you, of course. The present I told you she asked me to make sure you found and used."

"No, I haven't worn it yet."

Her look was outgoing, friendly. "Look, I know Mrs. Acton will be disappointed if you *don't* wear it. I'll bet the first thing she asks when she gets here on the weekend will be if you liked the bikini, *and* our beach."

"Mrs. Acton is definitely coming this weekend, then?" I'd been wondering about that.

"Mrs. Hacha says so. She was talking about it at breakfast, planning the weekend meals and such. That's why she wanted Adrian to go to town." She shook her head. "Didn't you know she was coming for the weekend?"

She said that as though it explained my bad manners in not trying out the bikini.

"She said she was," I admitted. "But Mrs. Acton is a very busy woman."

"She'll be here. And she'll ask you about the bikini—you can bet on it," she said, gathering my empty dishes. "Why don't you try it out right now? I would. While the sun's shining. You can be back before lunch. No problem. Why don't you, while Adrian is away? He has a thing about girls on beaches, and he can be a nuisance. Believe me, I know!"

I'll bet you do! I thought, but left it at that, without answering.

"If you happen to like it down there and are late for dinner, I'll tell Mrs. Hacha where you are," she said at the door. "That's one thing she has some sympathy about. She likes swimming even more than we do."

"I'll think about it," I said. "How does a person get down?"

"You can see where the steps start down from your window. Just walk across the lawns. I do. Make the most of the sun when it shines, *I* say. If I get the chance, I'll be down there with you."

She smiled and closed the door. Crockery

rattled faintly on her tray as she walked toward the stairs. I hesitated, frowning, thinking about what she'd said. She was right about one thing—I should try on the bikini. The tags were still on it up there in my drawer. She must've noticed, cleaning the room. And Vanessa would ask me how I liked the beach. Curiosity led me to the window to stare out and down, and I was lost.

Blue sea and a clean beach tempted me. I could almost feel the saltwater down there laving my body as I swam, renewing my energy, washing away the disappointment at not hearing from Paul or his mother. I'd work better for it, I knew. After all, part of the reason for my being here was for a vacation, which Vanessa had stressed.

The bikini fitted me like a second skin. I'd have to watch the sun, I knew. Only the shadow of a former suntan remained. I hadn't seen my skin as white in years. And Vanessa was right, the color of the bikini did flatter me, I decided. I found sandals and towel and was on my way.

The path down was not as bad as it looked from my window. There were slanting paths with steps as the way zigzagged down. It would be harder climbing back, but going down was painless. I looked around curiously as I stepped from the last concrete step onto the sand.

From where I stood, I couldn't see the great house on the clifftop above me. As Vanessa had said, it was like having your own beach on some lonely Pacific island. The only signs of civilization were a small shelter shed and the concrete steps themselves. I smiled and spread my towel on the beach, then decided against sunbathing and walked in up to my ankles in a sea that felt just cool enough to be refreshing. I couldn't resist it. I splashed out to my knees in water so clear I could see the grains of sand ahead. Deepening water, a small wave rolling in across flat sea, enticed me farther out.

I dived beneath the modest breaker, feeling it take hold of my body briefly, shake me, and then roll on past. Delighted, I tossed the water from my hair, and, turning, swam along the beach just outside the break. I swam slowly, getting the feel of it again. I swam level with the shelter shed, then turned and swam back faster, enjoying every moment of it.

Even if I came out of the water at once, I knew now, I would feel the better for this. This was my favorite sport. This was what my coming here was all about. Vanessa had sensed this. Thank you, Vanessa, I thought gratefully. I turned over on my back and closed my eyes, floating as I had been taught to do as a little girl. Already I could feel my tensions, soothed by the calm sea, beginning to fade.

Floating, I realized there was a current here, moving me insidiously into deeper water. But that did not worry me. I had no fear of a calm sea like this. I had regained confidence in my ability to swim out of any situation likely to arise.

I opened my eyes. I could see Finisterre now

quite clearly. I was right about the current. It had taken me a hundred yards out from where I had been swimming parallel to the beach. But I saw no problem in that. I could still swim back easily enough, even if I was out of training.

I was smiling and about to close my eyes again and give myself up to the soothing sensation of floating on calm waters when I caught the glint of sunlight on glass high up beneath the roof of Finisterre. I stared, puzzling as the glint came again and again, as whatever it was moved slightly beneath parted draperies. That was the fifth floor of the great house, I saw now, remembering that Sara Sheridan had told me the floors above mine were unoccupied. Wasted, Sara called it, for she could not understand how houses like this could have empty floors, the furniture swathed in protective sheets, when so many young people could not find even a tiny apartment that they could afford.

But if nobody lived up there, what was someone doing up there now, peering down at the sea from between stealthily parted draperies? Someone, something spying, moving, glinting. . . ?

I remembered Adrian suddenly, but Adrian was in Pescadero. Someone, though, was up there staring down at the sea. *Or at me?* The answer to that glinting sunlight came to me suddenly. Binoculars! Someone on the top floor of Finisterre was spying on me, watching me through field glasses. But why?

I began to feel angry suddenly, resenting those spying eyes! After all, there weren't many choices in deciding who that was. Adrian was in town, Pancho came into the house only when he was helping Adrian carry the library supplies upstairs. That had to be one of three women up there. Mrs. Hacha, or Jane Buchan, or Sara? So far as I knew, though, only Jane Buchan had reason to suspect I was not in the library.

But I realized suddenly then that someone else did know I was down here. Sara had appeared at the gate above the steps and was staring down at me incredulously. As I watched, she began to behave strangely. She was beckoning, and screaming at me in what was so obviously fright that I found myself becoming frightened too. And while I turned over, treading water as I tried to see her better, she began to run frenziedly down the steps toward me.

She was coming down so fast that she fell on the steep path, tumbling over and over while I stared in horror, expecting her to roll over the edge and fall to her death or serious injury. She was hurt, I could see. She got up slowly, still screaming and beckoning for me to come out. Raising myself in the water, I tried to hear.

"Come out, Samantha! *Come out!*"

As frightened as she was now, I started back in. I began to realize as I started swimming that I had been carried out much farther than I thought. It was a good two hundred yards to the beach, and the current taking me out was

much stronger than it had been. Momentarily I
was scared as I felt the strength of the water. I
started to swim harder, in fright, but forced
myself to be calm, to think. What you were
supposed to do when caught in a current like
this, I knew, was not to fight it but to let it take
you out, then turn and come in somewhere
away from the current.

But here, I saw now, that just wasn't possible. Let it take me *where*? On either side
were the cliffs, with their feet in deep water,
and between was this current that held me,
barely moving, even though I was swimming
strongly. If I let it sweep me out to sea, what
then? There was nothing but cliffs on either
side of the inlet that held Finisterre beach. I
had seen that in the car coming here with
Vanessa's chauffeur.

I mustn't panic! There was no place to go except the beach. I began to use greater power
with legs and arms, not rushing it but using all
my strength in stroking the way I had in distance racing. Gradually I began to realize that
I was moving toward the beach. The beach
crept closer despite the insidious strength of
the water. My forward movement increased
with the shallowing water. The sand was just
ahead. My feet found bottom, but my knees,
weakening, bent, and I scrambled awkwardly
from the water, panting.

With my breathing easing, I picked up my
towel. Sara had stopped where she was, halfway down. She was rubbing her knee and crying, I saw as I hurried to help her. I

remembered the watcher at the window, but could not see the house from where I was. I remembered vaguely glancing up as I reached shallow water. There had been movement up there as someone drew the draperies together.

"Sara," I called breathlessly. "Are you all right?"

"I bumped my knee, that's all." She started crying again as I climbed toward her. "I saw you from the kitchen window! *I didn't know what to do!* I couldn't find Mrs. Hacha or Jane. I was sure you'd drown! Didn't they tell you you can't swim down here when the tide's running out? You have to know the time the tide turns; there's a tide chart in the library. In a few more minutes you would have been swept out to sea. It's starting to run *now!* Look at it!"

I stared back and shivered. I could not have swum against the riptide I saw now. I didn't know anyone who could. A turmoil of water was frothing as it fought its way out to sea against small breakers coming in, thrusting them aside, breaking them prematurely, distorting them.

5

It was midafternoon when Adrian came into the library, his face flushed and angry. I looked up from the heap of books I was studying and sorting for subject matter to stare at him curiously. I'd become absorbed in the work. I'd recovered from what effort it had taken to get back to the beach, and the water had refreshed me. Sara wasn't hurt other than sore muscles and some minor bruises. Everyone who swims in the sea gets an occasional fright, but when the situation passes, it's over. You don't hate the sea for it, you just remember not to allow yourself to get caught in the same situation again.

I wasn't connecting Adrian's flushed face with what had happened to me as I asked innocently, "Is something the matter, Adrian?"

He shook his head, his face grim. "Sara just told me how she hurt herself this morning. She said after I left you went down to the beach and were almost taken out by the rip. Why did you do a thing like that? Didn't Mrs. Acton tell you about the riptide?"

"Would she know about it? She hasn't been here since her husband bought Finisterre, not until the last few days."

He frowned. "Mrs. Acton told you that?"

"Yes, she did. So I'm sure she didn't *know* about the tides. She would have warned me if she had."

"You were working when I left," he muttered. "It never occurred to me that you'd pick that tide to go swimming. It's my fault. I should have warned you."

I smiled affectionately at his obvious distress. "It wasn't anyone's *fault*, Adrian. Don't blame yourself for my ignorance about the danger of a riptide. It won't happen again. Sara says there's a tide chart in here. Next time, I'll check the tide before I swim."

His expression said that wasn't enough. "You must never swim there alone," he said grimly. "Others who have, drowned there on the ebb tide. If you had stayed in the water a few more minutes, you would be dead now. You can be sure of that, Miss Walton. Sara's call saved your life."

I shivered involuntarily. "Surely it's not as bad as that?" I muttered.

"I can't understand how you got back, as it was," he said. "You must have had the strength of desperation. Sara said the tide had already turned before she called you. She could see you being swept out. I don't know any other woman who could have got back to the beach.

My mother is a fine swimmer, and she couldn't. I know that!"

I shrugged. "It's over now, Adrian. I got back, thanks to Sara. Perhaps the danger wasn't as great as she thought. She was . . . excited."

"Mr. Acton died on a tide like it," he said. "The Actons should have warned you."

I stared at him, shocked. "Mr. Acton *drowned* down there?"

"On the beginning of an ebb tide, as you almost did!" he told me grimly. "Didn't the Actons tell you that?"

"Vanessa . . . Mrs. Acton said his death was the result of an accident. She didn't say where or how it happened. It distresses her talking about it, so I didn't ask questions. It never occurred to me that he *drowned here!*"

"There were others before him. Sick people. People trying to escape from Finisterre, people who saw the beach and the sea as a way to escape. Like Mr. Acton, their bodies were never found either. The bodies of people drowned here are never found. The action of the riptides and the currents in the outside reefs see to that. They wash beneath the reef among the giant kelp that grows outside. The kelp or the rocks hold them until sea creatures and decay destroy them and there's nothing left to float. The only chance would be the caves."

He had broken off abruptly. Still interested, I said, "Caves, you said? What caves?"

"There are caves with an entrance beneath the water under the southern headland," he said reluctantly. "A natural underwater tunnel leads into them. On the ebb tide a whirlpool forms above the entrance to the tunnel, and anything floating or swimming close to the southern cliff to come within reach of the maelstrom is sucked down and through the tunnel into the outer cave."

I shuddered, remembering suddenly that I had thought of allowing the ebb tide to take me that way, intending to find some rock above the tide level and try to climb on it.

"How horrible!" I muttered, thinking about what might have happened.

"The caves are beautiful," he said defensively. "The sea formed and smoothed them, and it cleanses them by the rise and fall of the tides. They are dry except when the big tides come, and even then they're safe, for the air inside is pure. There must be cracks in the rock crevices somewhere that keep the air fresh. But there's no way any ordinary swimmer could make it through the tunnel alive."

I stared at him. "Yet you speak as though you've been in there?"

Momentarily he glanced at me, startled, either by the realization of what he had said or by my question. I was not sure which.

"I found the tunnel when I was searching for Mr. Acton's body," he said. "I was wearing scuba gear."

"He . . . wasn't down there?"

"No." He glanced as though returning to the present from some unpleasant memory. "Are

you sorting the books already? I could help you
with that, save time . . . ?"

But I was not prepared to let him escape my
curiosity yet. I decided to appeal to his vanity.

"You dived into this awful tunnel? Not
knowing what was inside, or even whether you
could turn around and swim back out again?
That was a brave thing you did, Adrian.
Weren't you afraid? Were you alone down
there? Please tell me about it. The books can
wait."

He moved uneasily, embarrassed. "I was nervous the first time, yes," he said slowly. "It was
night, and though I had a light, it was . . .
weird down there. But it was safe. By the time
we missed Mr. Acton and realized what must
have happened, the tide was turning to come
back in. I only had one bad moment when the
Aqua-lung cylinder almost got stuck at a place
where the tunnel narrowed. I had to turn on
my side to make it."

I shuddered sympathetically. "I would've
died of fright down there under the sea in the
night!"

"I've never used the Aqua-lung there since.
All anyone really needs is a face mask and
snorkel tube. It's perfectly safe if you choose
the right tide and know what you're doing, and
I do." He hesitated. "I've taken my mother and
other people down there. It's quite a place. I
could show it to you, if you like. When the
tide's right."

"No thanks!" I said hastily.

"I wouldn't ask you to do anything if there

was any danger to you in doing it," he declared indignantly.

"I know that, Adrian," I told him quickly. "It's just that . . . Well, I like swimming, but underwater exploration doesn't appeal to me."

"The inlet was my playground when I was a little boy," he said, appeased. "I know every hazard down there. Every reef, every kelp bed. I know where the lobsters live, and the big fish. Anytime my mother wants fish for the kitchen, I can get all she wants in half an hour with a speargun."

I smiled, amused at what I thought his conceit. "I'll bet you can, Adrian!"

He frowned. "I wasn't boasting, Miss Walton. What I was trying to say was that if you swim down there again and I know, you'll be quite safe. I mean, I'd watch over your safety even if I wasn't in the water. I wouldn't be a nuisance, or bother you in any way by swimming with you. Not unless you asked me to. But if I knew you were going to the beach, I wouldn't worry. I wouldn't be scared stiff on sunny days about what you might do. Is it too much to ask that you just . . . let me know when you feel like swimming?"

Touched by his anxiety, I smiled involuntarily. "I promise I won't go swimming again without letting you know, Adrian. If you do want to swim at the same time, that wouldn't bother me. Why should it?"

After all, who else was there at Finisterre I could go swimming with? Sara had told me this morning as I helped her back from the beach that *she* was no swimmer, and rarely did more than sunbathe there, or paddle on the edge. And as swimming companions, both Adrian's mother and Jane Buchan were out as far as I was concerned.

That left only Vanessa and Paul. I became aware that Adrian was speaking to me, and that he looked as though what I'd said had made his day.

"One day I'll take you down to my cave," he was saying. "You'll realize how safe it is and want to come in when I show you the tunnel."

Already he was becoming possessive again. I frowned. "I doubt it, Adrian." I looked down at my work again. "Now, suppose you find me anything we can file under the subject of anthropology. I'll check them out, and we'll stack them apart as candidates for the one-to-one-hundred group."

"Will you tell me something first? Something about this morning that's worrying me?"

I shook my head at him, smiling. "Really, Adrian, that's all over and done with! It can't happen again now that I know about the tides, and I've promised I won't go swimming without letting you know. So, shall we go back to work? Mrs. Acton will expect some progress made when she gets here on the weekend."

"This is . . . very important to me, Miss Walton," he pleaded, his brown eyes appealing.

"Well . . . don't make it too long. What is it?"

"What prompted you to go rushing down there the moment I left? You hadn't mentioned swimming. You hadn't even looked out the window at the beach, or seemed to notice what kind of day it was. What was your *reason* for suddenly wanting to swim?"

I frowned, considering. "Did I have to have a reason? I remember looking at the sun on the beach. I hadn't wanted to go until then, not even when Jane Buchan reminded me Mrs. Acton had left me a bikini for a present and I hadn't used it yet."

"*Jane Buchan* reminded you about a bikini Mrs. Acton gave you? *Jane?*" He was studying my face intently, anxiously, I thought.

"Mrs. Acton bought it for me and left it in my bedroom, together with a note welcoming me to Finisterre," I explained. "She asked Jane to make sure I found it, and Jane did." I glanced around. "Only, then I began to get interested in what we're doing here. I forgot the bikini."

"Until *Jane* reminded you?"

"I hadn't thought about it until then. No."

"Didn't she say anything about the tide?" he asked angrily.

"No. I suppose she forgot. She didn't know I *would* take her advice. I didn't *say* I would. But when she parted the draperies and I saw the sunshine and the blue sea, I was tempted. I *like* swimming. I thought: why not?"

"*She knows how dangerous the ebb tide can be!*"

Something odd in his voice made me look at him more closely, and I saw to my surprise that his brown eyes had narrowed, glinting with a cold fury.

"I don't believe she thought about the tides, Adrian," I said in the girl's defense. "I don't blame Jane for what happened. She only reminded me about the bikini and that when Mrs. Acton comes here she will be sure to ask me if I like it, and what I think of the beach. Mrs. Acton is proud of Finisterre, even if she had reason not to come here since Mr. Acton's death." I could understand her reason for that better now. Thanks to Adrian.

"The tide chart is over there between the two windows," he said coldly. "Jane could have seen it wherever she stood in this room. And there is another one like it in the kitchen that the staff must look at before they go swimming."

"*I* never noticed it before."

I was looking at it now, though. The chart for today said quite plainly that there was a high tide of five feet, one inch at eleven A.M. Jane had brought up morning coffee a little after ten-thirty. Adrian left, I had coffee, changed, and walked down to the sea. The tide would have just turned, just started to run out as I reached the beach. Thought of that made me feel sick suddenly. There had been a lot of water to run out from that five-feet-one-inch high tide!

"There was no reason why you should," Adrian's voice said harshly. "But before you came, Jane and I met in here for morning coffee. We'd look at the chart together to see if

Simply put, they're as low as you can go and still get good taste.

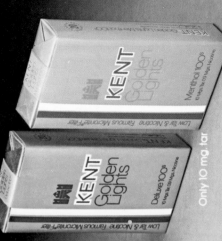

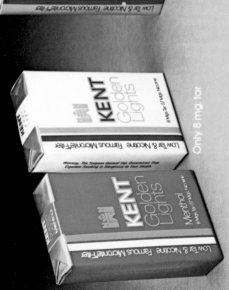

Only 10 mg. tar

Only 8 mg. tar

Kent Golden Lights 100's Regular and Menthol: 10 mg. "tar," 0.9 mg. nicotine.
Kings Menthol: 8 mg. "tar," 0.7 mg. nicotine av. per cigarette by FTC Method.
Kings Regular: 8 mg. "tar," 0.6 mg. nicotine av. per cigarette FTC Report April 1977.

Warning: The Surgeon General Has Determined That Cigarette Smoking Is Dangerous to Your Health.

Compare your brand with Kent Golden Lights

FILTER BRANDS (KING SIZE)

REGULAR	MG TAR	MG NIC	MENTHOL	MG TAR	MG NIC
Kent Golden Lights Kings	8	0.6	Kent Golden Lights Menthol*	8	0.7
Real*	9	0.8	Real Menthol*	9	0.8
Parliament*	10	0.8	Vantage Menthol	11	0.7
Vantage Kings	10	0.7	Salem Lights	11	0.8
Marlboro Lights	13	0.8	Doral Menthol	11	0.8
Winston Lights	13	0.9	Kool Milds	14	0.9
Doral	13	0.9	Belair	15	1.0
Viceroy Kings	16	1.0	Kool	17	1.3
Tareyton Kings*	16	1.2	Salem	18	1.2
Marlboro Kings	18	1.1			
Winston Kings	19	1.2			

*FTC Method

FILTER BRANDS (100's)

REGULAR	MG TAR	MG NIC	MENTHOL	MG TAR	MG NIC
Kent Golden Lights 100's*	10	0.9	Kent Golden Lights Menthol 100's*	10	0.9
Vantage 100's*	11	0.9	Merit Menthol 100's*	12	0.9
Merit 100's*	12	0.9	Salem Long Lights*	12	0.9
Parliament 100's*	12	0.9	Virginia Slims	16	0.9
Winston Lights 100's*	14	1.0	Menthol 100's	16	0.9
Virginia Slims 100's*	16	1.0	Benson & Hedges Menthol 100's	18	1.0
Tareyton 100's*	16	1.2	Salem 100's	18	1.2
Benson & Hedges 100's*	18	1.0	Belair 100's	18	1.3
Marlboro 100's	18	1.1	Kool 100's	18	1.3
Pall Mall Gold 100's	19	1.4	Winston Menthol 100's	19	1.2

*FTC Method

Kent Golden Lights
Taste 'em. You won't believe the numbers.

Kent Golden Lights

Of All Brands Sold: Lowest tar: 0.5 mg. "tar," 0.05 mg. nicotine av. per cigarette, FTC Report, December 1976. **Kent Golden Lights 100's Regular and Menthol:** 10 mg. "tar," 0.9 mg. nicotine. **Kings Menthol:** 8 mg. "tar," 0.7 mg. nicotine av. per cigarette by FTC Method. **Kings Regular:** 8 mg. "tar," 0.6 mg. nicotine av. per cigarette FTC Report, April 1977.

it was okay to swim at lunchtime. Such things become a habit. Jane knew the chart was there, Miss Walton. She knew that very well."

I shrugged. "People forget, Adrian," I reminded him.

"Without checking the tide, she influenced you to go down there," he said. "*Alone!* When *she* knows how dangerous it can be. *I can't get that out of my mind!*"

I managed to smile and suggest: "The best way to do that is to start collecting some anthropology books for me, Adrian. Okay?"

He muttered something and went to work. After that we didn't speak of it again. Sara limped in with coffee halfway through the afternoon. She said Jane was in her room, when Adrian asked.

"Sulking!" she confided to me with a slightly malicious smile, when Adrian was out of hearing. "Mrs. Hacha finally decided to let me have this weekend off. I feel guilty, though. She's expecting Mrs. Acton down for the weekend. They will be busy."

"Just enjoy your weekend, Sara," I told her, smiling. "So far as I'm concerned, you've certainly earned it!" I remembered Paul was coming down too, but neglected to mention that.

Days passed quickly, for Adrian and I were beginning to see something for our work now as the first section of shelves cleared and books cataloged under anthropology and autobiography began to be cleaned and shelved in their places. Adrian's help, I had to admit, was invaluable. So was his memory for books that he had read or noticed, and their subject matter.

Almost before I realized it, it was Friday evening.

I looked around with satisfaction after Adrian had left me alone in the library to gather some material I wanted to check in my room. The anthropology-subject-matter books were finished, cleaned, repaired, and numbered. Their cards were filed in the cabinet. It was time, I decided proudly, to give Vanessa at least a progress report, since she had refrained from contacting me all week.

At least, that was the excuse I made myself for wanting to talk to Vanessa, when I knew she would be coming to see me next day. Because, I admitted secretly, I longed for the conversation of someone closer to me personally than Mrs. Hacha and the servants, even poor Sara. Maybe Vanessa and I were not that close yet, but if she was to become my mother-in-law, I could expect she would be.

With my mind made up to call Vanessa, the day seemed even better. The uneasy doubts in my mind, that because I hadn't heard from Vanessa all week, she might not be coming, would be put at rest. And of course she would reassure me that Paul was coming with her, and explain why Paul hadn't called me either.

With these thoughts I went happily downstairs to ask Mrs. Hacha for Vanessa's Bel Air telephone number and which telephone I could use to call. I found the housekeeper in the kitchen working with a sullen-looking Jane

Buchan, who barely raised her eyes to look at me and at once went off into the laundry as though she had urgent work to do elsewhere, closing the dividing door behind her.

I discovered Mrs. Hacha looking at me as though I had no business in her kitchen and she resented the interruption of my presence. "Well?" she asked tartly.

I managed to smile. "I thought I should ask you about calling Mrs. Acton in Bel Air. I want to report progress. Adrian and I have done quite well."

"I thought Mrs. Acton told you she's coming down tomorrow."

"Yes, she did. But I haven't heard from her all week. Or from my fiancé." Because her tone angered me, I asked her bluntly: "Which telephone should I use? And can you tell me her number?"

Her lips thinned, and she frowned at me. "Mrs. Acton called the telephone company when she was here last weekend, because the line is faulty. We can't send or receive long-distance calls. They haven't sent a repairman. I doubt you could get through if you tried, so why not wait until tomorrow?"

She had turned back to the list she was checking, as though that ended the matter, and for the moment I stared at her blankly. "No long-distance calls? Is that why Mrs. Acton hasn't phoned me? She can't get through?"

"Of course," she said.

"My mother hasn't noticed the time, Miss Walton. It's after business hours, and long-distance calls are easier to make now. If you like, I could get Mrs. Acton's home for you on the phone in the living room. It's quite private for you in there."

Adrian had come in unnoticed by his mother, who was staring at him in startled disbelief. "What makes you think you know more than anyone else about our telephones?" she demanded furiously.

"Because I've often called Bel Air for you in off-peak hours and got through. Remember?" His expressionless face turned toward me. "Want me to try for you, Miss Walton?" He added for his mother's benefit, "I'm sure Mrs. Acton will be pleased when you tell her what we've done this week."

I wanted to say yes, but undermining Mrs. Hacha's authority wasn't anything I wanted to do. I hadn't come to Finisterre to make her an enemy. I looked at her inquiringly.

"Go on," she said disgustedly. "Let him try, Miss Walton."

To placate her, I asked politely, "If Adrian does get through, would you like to speak to Mrs. Acton, Mrs. Hacha? I could ask her to hold the line."

"We can discuss our housekeeping problems when she gets here tomorrow," she said resentfully. "So don't bother, *if* you get Mrs. Acton."

Having made the gesture, I followed Adrian along the passage to the living room, a room I hadn't been in before. It was large enough to be the reception room of a Renaissance palace, but it was furnished with the heavy, leather-covered furniture of the turn of the century. The leather was well worn, and the room smelled faintly of dust and disuse, and needed airing. Glancing around, I saw the bars at the windows and wondered who had filled those leather chairs and lounges, patients or staff. I supposed Adrian would know.

"It's only during the day that we have trouble with the line. Long-distance calls are impossible most of the time then," Adrian said apologetically. In defense, I knew, of his mother.

"That's probably why I haven't heard from Mrs. Acton or my fiancé."

"I would think so. Mrs. Acton usually forgets and tries to call Finisterre during the day. I don't know about Paul. He's never phoned here that I know of. The Acton phone number in Bel Air is in this book. But I know it well. Shall I try?"

"Please do, Adrian."

Waiting, I imagined Vanessa answering, and what I would say. Was Paul well? Why hadn't he called? Was Paul . . . ?

"I think we're getting through," Adrian said encouragingly. "Takes a little time. An impatient person could hang up and stop trying. I wait. Is your fiancé an impatient type?"

"In some ways," I said, remembering.

"Mrs. Acton and my mother are quite good friends. Did you know that?"

"No, not really. In what way?"

"Not as just housekeeper and mistress," he said. "I mean real friends. They've known each other for a long time. Before Mother began to work for her."

"I didn't know *that*," I admitted, surprised.

"I'm getting through," he said. "You take it now. I'll go back to the kitchen."

"Mrs. Acton's residence," a woman's voice said.

I took the phone, hearing him close the door. "This is Miss Walton calling from Finisterre. Can I speak to Mrs. Acton, please?"

"Mrs. Acton isn't at home this evening. Can I take a message?"

"Is Paul there?"

"Mr. Acton has been away all week. I understand he isn't coming home this weekend. I can give either of them a message when they do come home."

"When are you expecting Mrs. Acton home?"

"She didn't say. Perhaps if you call in the morning?"

"I'll wait until I see her here at Finisterre."

"I'll tell Mrs. Acton you called."

There was something odd about the woman's voice. Evasiveness? Embarrassment? I couldn't put a name to it.

I thanked her and hung up, feeling frustrated. I decided Paul must be coming straight through to San Francisco from Phoenix. That was why he wasn't expected home at Bel Air. Vanessa would meet him at the airport, and they'd drive down to Finisterre together. Satisfied with my reasoning, I still felt the need to talk to someone I liked. I thought of Anne Amberg, back in Palo Alto. I glanced at the clock ōn the wall. Anne should be having dinner at home before leaving for the library. She should have returned from the short vacation she'd planned and be starting work again tonight.

If I phoned the apartment superintendent, Mrs. Pettit, she would call Anne, and Anne could take the call in Mrs. Pettit's office. There had been plans to install phones in the apartments for two years, but it had never been done. Most of us didn't mind. We used Mrs. Pettit's phone and paid for our calls as we made them, or walked to the phone booth at the corner drugstore. This was better than getting phone bills anyway. Our low rentals more than balanced any inconvenience, most of us thought.

I knew the apartment-building telephone number by heart, and if Adrian could put a call through to Los Angeles, I should be able to call Palo Alto. I got through even more easily than Adrian had. But the voice that answered me was a man's voice, not Mrs. Pettit's rather squeaky mezzo-soprano.

"Who is that?" I demanded, puzzling.

"Carter, miss. I'm the new janitor."

"Could I speak to Mrs. Pettit, please?" A janitor? I frowned.

"I'm sorry, miss, but I don't know any Mrs. Pettit here."

"Mrs. Pettit is the super."

"Mr. Smith is the super."

"*Mrs. Pettit* is the superintendent," I said, exasperated. "I should know, I *live* there."

"Wait. Mrs. Pettit, you said? Was she the lady who used to work for the Methodists?"

"What do you mean, *used to* work for them?" I demanded irritably. "Isn't Mrs. Pettit there anymore?"

"Not since last week, when the building changed hands. You must be one of the girls who went home on vacation when the college closed for the summer. Didn't you know the apartment building has been sold?"

"I certainly did not!" I said, shocked.

"It was sudden," he admitted. "They said a lot of the girls who lived here haven't been notified yet. There wasn't time. Is there anything *I* can do for you, miss? I can't get you Mr. Smith, as he's in the city."

"I wanted to talk to Miss Anne Amberg. She lives in apartment nineteen. Mrs. Pettit used to take phone calls for the tenants. She'd let us use her office phone. If you could ask Miss Amberg to come to the phone, I'd be most grateful."

"You're going to find some changes here when you come back, miss," the janitor said conversationally. "We've had technicians working nonstop all week. A lot of the apartments have had phones installed. Just wait till I check! Yes, I can put you through directly to apartment nineteen. Hold the line."

I heard the phone ring at the other end in Anne's apartment. After a while a reluctant male voice said, "Hello?"

The voice was loud; it had to be to make itself heard above a background of laughter, music, and high-pitched conversation. It sounded as though Anne was throwing a party and everyone was having a ball. The male voice must mean we could now have *men* visit us in the apartments. As the janitor said, things had indeed changed.

"Could I speak to Miss Amberg, please?"

"*Miss who?*"

"Miss Amberg. *Anne Amberg*," I shouted back. "That's her apartment you're in!" And good luck to you, Anne, I thought. Anyway, why not have a party if you want one. And the guy had a nice voice. It was the summer vacation, wasn't it?

"Anne? I don't know any Anne here right now. Look, why don't you come up and join us? Then you can find Anne for yourself, if she's here. I don't know a lot of these people, *yet*. We're all too new here. What did you say your name was?"

"I'm Samantha Walton. I lease the next apartment, twenty-one, but right now I'm calling long distance. I'm in a beach house near Pescadero. So don't be long, *please?*"

"What makes you think Anne What's-her-name is here?" he asked petulantly.

"I told you," I said patiently. "That's Anne's apartment you're in."

"That's funny! I thought that was what you said the first time. You think *this* is her apartment?"

"I've lived next door to her there for *three years*," I said. "Please, just call Anne for me. Long-distance calls cost, remember."

"Wait!" he said dramatically. "I see light! The noise you hear is the housewarming. I only moved in yesterday. If Anne was the previous tenant, she moved out last Monday."

"But that's impossible!" I cried, shocked. "Where would she *go*? You just can't get apartments as cheap as those anywhere in Palo Alto!"

"You can't get an *apartment* anywhere in this town! Period!" he said. "I know! As for these being the cheapest apartments in Palo Alto—if they once were, that isn't so now. These *cost*! But that's the name of the game. People don't buy places like this unless they can see a profit in it. Some LA realtors bought it, and took over management right away."

"To throw out people like Anne and I who have lived there for three years or more!" I said indignantly.

"Well, little as I like speculators," he said, "I have to admit that's not quite right. Your tenant friends who have gone, went of their own free will."

"I'll bet!"

"No, *really*," he said. "They did. Prompted, we've heard, by quite a generous compensation for relinquishing their leases." He broke off abruptly to yell: "Hey, watch it! That's new carpet!" He came back on to say hurriedly, "Look, I'll have to go! Things are getting a bit out of hand!"

"Can you tell me the name of the realtors? I'd better check on what they're doing about my apartment, if it still is mine."

But he had already gone.

I put the phone down slowly and went upstairs to my room, with all my problems still unsolved, and the added worry of whether I could keep my apartment or not.

6

Although my work in Vanessa's library was running smoothly, I seemed to be frustrated everywhere else. I called Bel Air twice on Saturday morning, but the same woman answered and gave the same replies. No, Mrs. Acton wasn't home. She hadn't heard from her since the last time I called. Mr. Acton wasn't home either. So far as she knew, they were still both coming to Finisterre for the weekend. At least, if they were not, neither Mrs. Acton nor Paul had advised her otherwise, or left any message for me in case I called.

When I called the second time, relations between us seemed to have become a little strained. She told me brusquely that there was no change whatever in the situation from when I phoned earlier. She almost hung up on me impatiently when I said I was sorry to be giving her so much trouble, phoning—but I was worried about them both.

"There's nothing for *anyone* to be worried about," she told me disgustedly just before she put her phone down. "Mrs. Acton is inclined to be careless about confiding her movements to *anyone*. She's the mistress, so she comes and goes as she pleases. She could walk into Finisterre any moment now, or she may not come at all. Mr. Paul is more predictable than his mother—unless they're together. And they probably *are*, you know. . . ."

I put down the phone disconsolately as she hung up, and went miserably back upstairs. I had told Adrian Hacha he need not work in the library over the weekend, but he had smiled and started work. He had nothing else interesting to do, he said. I was glad that he had come to work. I needed company, and he knew it.

I fidgeted, unable to work efficiently, alternating between the shelves and the window each time I fancied I heard a car driving in. But the slow day passed without any sign of Vanessa or Paul. I had made up my mind not to call Bel Air again that day, but when I closed the library with darkness falling outside, it took effort not to try again.

What was the use? I asked myself finally as I went upstairs to prepare for my meal, waited on alone in the dining room. Vanessa and Paul wouldn't be going back to Bel Air. They were coming directly to Finisterre. There was nowhere that I knew of, other than the Bel Air house, where I *could* call them. I had to be patient, to wait. Paul would come. Nobody could keep Paul away. We hadn't seen each other for almost *two weeks!* If he didn't come today, he would tomorrow.

The trouble was, I wanted Paul to come *to-day!*

I sat in the living room after dinner, sipping coffee and trying to read the notes I'd made on the suggestions Vanessa's professor friend had left me. I tried, but my mind wasn't on it. My mind was on the road from San Francisco International Airport. But although I checked continually for the gleam of headlights coming through the forest, there was no sign of Ed Hart and the Acton limousine.

In the end I went miserably up to bed, feeling more rejected even than I'd felt when my parents' marriage broke up and I discovered that because of their new interests neither of them wanted me.

I slept badly and wakened with a headache and that dull feeling of frustration and anxiety that follows a sleepless night. I'd left the draperies apart so that I might see the headlights if Vanessa and Paul arrived late at night. They had not.

Even the bright sunlight streaming in after a perfect fogless night could not make me feel better. I'd slept late when at last I fell asleep, and now there was barely enough time to shower and dress for breakfast. Jane Buchan hadn't brought me any coffee this morning, an omission that I was sure was deliberate. Whatever she had to do for me in the course of her work now, she performed reluctantly or not at all. Getting ready for breakfast, I lost my taste for it, remembering that Jane would be on duty downstairs again this morning.

I was going to have to do something about Jane Buchan if she persisted in being unreasonably jealous just because Adrian was working with me in the library. Or maybe her open hostility toward me now had another reason? Adrian had been furious about her behavior on the day I went swimming on an ebb tide. I suspected he'd attacked her about that, although he hadn't mentioned it to me.

Several times I intended to tell Jane Buchan that I hadn't blamed *her* for what happened. Only, Adrian had done that. I knew it couldn't have been deliberate. And in any case, I was quite able to take care of myself in the water, even against a riptide like the one that had been building as I swam out. If there was fault in my blundering into danger through ignorance of local conditions, I couldn't blame anyone but myself.

I wanted to tell her these things, but she was so surly, so openly hostile and unapproachable, that each time I had the impulse, her sullen, angry expression turned me away. She just wasn't the kind of girl you could reason with.

It was the same this sunny Sunday morning. She served the fruit juice and the cereal without once raising her pale gray eyes to look at me.

"Mrs. Hacha says do you want your eggs poached, boiled, or fried with bacon?"

"Soft-boiled, please, and just one egg, not

two." She was turning away silently, her face sullen. I said, "Jane . . ."

She stopped to look at me warily. "Yes?"

"It would be much easier for both of us if we could be friends, don't you think so?"

"You know why we're not!" she said, her eyes suddenly full of hate. "You blamed *me* for sending you swimming down there on the ebb tide. You had to tell Adrian that, didn't you?"

"I told Adrian people forget such things. I didn't blame you, why should I? People don't do things like that *deliberately*. It was just an accident, and there was no harm done."

"Not to you!" She had raised her voice involuntarily. "But what about *me*?"

"I wouldn't have mentioned your name, but Adrian asked me why I went down there immediately after he had gone. He said if I'd even mentioned I might go swimming, he would have warned me not to." I shrugged. "I told him about the bikini Paul's mother left for me and that you reminded me I hadn't used it and Mrs. Acton would be sure to ask if I had, and what I thought of the beach."

"And *you* didn't think that would get me into trouble, I suppose?"

"I didn't see why it should." Suddenly, though, I remembered the gleam of sunlight on glass at one of the upstairs windows. "Someone was watching me through binoculars from the top floor of the house. I saw her when I was floating and lazing about in the water. Was that you?"

"Me?" she asked furiously. "If I had been,

wouldn't I have *noticed* you were being carried out? Is that what you meant to ask next? Well, for your information, I don't own any binoculars, Miss Walton! And I don't know anyone at Finisterre who does! I know Adrian doesn't, or Sara Sheridan, or Adrian's mother. And I'm not going to let you tell Adrian that it was me up there watching you. We're not allowed on that floor at any time. Those rooms are kept locked, and—"

"*Jane!*"

Mrs. Hacha had come into the room unnoticed and was standing watching us, her face expressionless.

Jane turned quickly, almost dropping her tray. "Yes, Mrs. Hacha?" she mumbled, as though in sudden fright. Her face had paled as she saw the housekeeper.

"When I ask you to take the breakfast order from Miss Walton, I expect you to come back with it in time for me to cook it for her!" the housekeeper said coldly.

"I was coming, when she stopped me!" she said with a vindictive glance in my direction. "She said—"

"I heard you being insolent to Miss Walton. I'll talk to you about that later. How does Miss Walton want her breakfast eggs?"

"Boiled, she said. But—"

"Boil them, then."

"But—"

"The way she wants them. *Now*, Jane. You hear me?" The housekeeper was studying her angrily. Jane gave me a furious look and fled.

"I have a message for you," Mrs. Hacha said, studying me with inscrutable black eyes. "Mrs. Acton phoned. She said to inform you she regrets she cannot come to Finisterre this weekend, but she will definitely be here for the following one."

I stared at her disbelievingly. "Why didn't she speak to me? Why just leave me a message? Was she at the airport or someplace where she couldn't wait?"

"She did not ask to speak to you, Miss Walton, because she phoned *me* very late last night. You had gone upstairs hours before, and she decided, and I agreed, that you would be fast asleep."

"Is Paul coming this weekend?" I demanded. "What did she say about Paul?"

She frowned at me, considering. "She didn't give me any message for you about her son, Miss Walton," she said slowly.

"You don't *know* whether Paul is coming here today or not? But she knows I'm expecting Paul. It was she who told me he would *be* here." The dark eyes in that arrogant face were hard to meet, but I held them angrily until she looked away. "Paul and I are engaged to be married, Mrs. Hacha," I reminded her.

She nodded. "So I was informed. Engaged, but not yet married. All I can tell you is that I was not instructed to prepare for Mr. Acton's coming. I don't believe I would expect that, if I were you. The last I heard, he was in Arizona assisting Mr. Harding in some disputed land claim before the court. Such procedures, I believe, drag on for weeks."

I stared at her blankly in dismay. *"Weeks?"*

"But no doubt if he's in love with you he will call you long distance to tell you about that himself. After all, Arizona, or wherever he is, is not the moon, Miss Walton. Why don't you go swimming and forget about it? Fretting never hastens or heals such things. I may go down to the beach myself. But as my son has told you— not on the ebb tide."

"I'm not likely to forget that."

She nodded. "You must be a very strong swimmer, Miss Walton. Sara Sheridan said the tide had already turned before she saw you. Yet you swam back against it?"

"Perhaps fear lent me strength, Mrs. Hacha."

She frowned. "Sheridan said you were floating happily on your back, basking. You must have felt the current taking you out."

"I did. But at that time, I knew I could swim back. Later, I wasn't so sure. What scared me was the way it strengthened so fast." I shook my head. "I won't be caught like that again."

"I heard you tell that stupid girl you saw someone watching you through binoculars from the top floor of the house. You asked if it was her, and she told you none of us have binoculars." She shook her head, studying my face. "She told the truth. None of us do. But I have seen what you saw."

"You think it was something different? *Not* the sun shining on the lenses?"

"I have seen it often," she said calmly. "I too

like to float about down there in the warm sun
and let the sea take me where it will. It *is* the
sun on glass, as you thought. On the window
glass between draperies not properly closed.
The window where you saw the reflection is the
third from the right, just under the eaves, isn't
it?"

I considered, frowning. "Yes, I think so.
Why?"

"The draperies are old and worn," she said.
"They do not close properly. Because they cannot close, the sunlight is reflected from the glass
between."

"But there was someone there. I saw the draperies close."

"You imagined you did," she said. "Or perhaps it was an optical illusion caused by the action of swimming so strongly. There was no one
up there, Miss Walton. That floor is locked,
sealed off. It hasn't been in use since the Actons
bought Finisterre. I suppose by now you have
learned that this house was once a mental hospital?"

"Yes."

"Servants have long tongues!" she said vin-
dictively. "That floor was used for the worst
cases. It was a grim place where people were
kept confined in maximum security, because
they could be extremely dangerous. It has not
been touched since. That is why it is kept
locked. Nobody could be up there. Unless the
ghost of some poor wretch who died there."

"But. . . ."

"There's no other explanation for what you

saw, Miss Walton." She glanced toward the kitchen. "That fool girl should have brought your eggs back long ago! Excuse me."

I watched her go, frowning. But I *had* seen someone up there! Someone who drew the draperies together?

Or had I?

I found I'd lost my appetite for the egg, even before it came, and I found that from spite Jane Buchan had boiled it so long the yolk was hard and tough. I wandered out into the garden after breakfast. The sun was still shining, the sea a fantastic blue. I found a garden seat and sat there deciding whether I should work in the library or rest today.

I decided on the library, as I remembered that Adrian might be there waiting to see whether I meant to work or not. Last night I'd been undecided. This morning I kept asking myself what else was there. I mean, whatever I did, I'd be road-watching most of the time, for I couldn't believe Paul wouldn't come. Paul wasn't like that. If something had come up to make it imperative that he stay on in Arizona, Paul would let me know. He wouldn't just leave me up in the air, worrying myself sick the way I was.

That was what worried me most, I admitted secretly. This neglect. If there was one thing Paul was not, it was inconsiderate.

I walked back across the untidy lawns to the house, meaning to enter, as I had left, by the dining-room door that opened onto a side porch. To my disgust, I found the door locked on the inside in my absence. Forced to walk back to the front entrance and wait Jane's pleasure in answering the bell, I saw her spite again in the locked door.

I rang the doorbell, expecting a long wait, but my ring was answered almost at once, the door opening.

"I didn't expect to see *you*, Samantha!" Adrian had answered the bell, not Jane Buchan. "I hoped it was Mrs. Acton or her son, knowing how worried you are. I thought you were still at breakfast."

"I finished early and went for a walk in the sunshine. Someone locked the dining-room door while I was outside."

"Jane?" he asked, frowning.

"I don't know who, or why. It's not important. I was trying to make up my mind whether to work today, or rest."

"I'll help out if you do—but I have a better idea."

I began to walk toward the library with him. "You have?"

"The sea is as calm as a pond today, and the tide is running in all morning. It's perfectly safe today, if you'd like to swim."

I frowned. "I hadn't thought about swimming, Adrian. But if you want to, remember, you don't have to work today."

"I can swim anytime," he said. "But you've been working hard for a long time, here and at college, and now you're worried about the Actons not coming. You are worried about them, aren't you?"

"That's why I thought I'd work," I admitted miserably. "But you don't have to."

"Neither do you, Miss Walton," he said anxiously. "How much work do you think you can do today? It will be like it was yesterday. You'll keep looking out the window and wondering where they are and why they haven't contacted you. You'll be too worried to work efficiently. You know that."

"Was I that obvious yesterday, Adrian?"

"I found myself worrying about you."

Touched by his obvious sympathy and sincerity, I smiled and gave in. He was right, I conceded. Yesterday there had been work I knew I had botched and would have to do again. And it would be the same today.

"What do you suggest we do, Adrian? Go down to the beach?"

"I told you once before that I'd never bother you, or be a nuisance by swimming when you are," he said quietly. "I just want to be where I can see that you're safe. To . . ." He hesitated, frowning. "To . . . protect you if you need that, I guess. That's all."

I smiled at his confusion. "As I remember it, you also said you wouldn't swim unless I wanted you to swim with me. And I replied that it wouldn't bother me if you did."

He looked up at me quickly. "You wouldn't mind if I swam with you today?"

"I think I need company. I know I wouldn't go swimming alone today. The way I feel, I couldn't enjoy it. I'll see you on the beach. Okay?"

When I glanced back as I started upstairs, he was standing outside the library door watching me. His expression gave me a feeling of guilt. It seemed to me Adrian was falling for me. Momentarily I was tempted to call our swim off, and looked back from the first stair, but found I could not.

"In about an hour," I said. "Okay?"

"Great!" he said exultantly.

I was longer upstairs than I meant to be. I called Bel Air again. A different woman answered. But she gave the same answers. Vanessa hadn't been home; neither had Paul. So far as she knew, they were still coming to Finisterre.

I walked slowly down the path and the steps to the beach, already regretting my decision to go swimming with Adrian, so miserable did I feel. Even the perfect day wasn't helping, and I felt worse when, as I descended the last few steps, I noticed the dark-haired girl sunbathing on a towel at the far end of the beach, her face on her arm, watching me. Jane Buchan!

Adrian was sprawled on a towel by himself close to the steps. He sat up as I reached the sand, and I noticed his wet trunks.

"It's great in," he said, smiling. "I think you'll enjoy it." He stood up. "Would you like to sunbathe first?"

"Isn't that Jane farther along the beach?"

He nodded. "Yes. I was swimming when she came down. She went over there while I was in the water."

"Why don't you call her back? We could sunbathe together."

"She wouldn't come," he said grimly. "She's in a bad mood this morning. Wouldn't even answer when I called her. She's like that."

"Because I'm here? I shouldn't have come!"

He looked his dismay. "Don't let her spoil your swim! I brought snorkels and flippers. I thought maybe you'd let me show you some of the things I've discovered among the reefs and in the kelp beds."

I looked along the beach at Jane Buchan uneasily. "I should go back to the house. The Actons could come."

"My mother thinks not," he said. "And she should know. Have you used a snorkel?" He added eagerly, "I could teach you in ten minutes."

"I learned when I was a little girl. We lived in Santa Monica." That had been in the good days, I remembered. Before my parents' marriage broke up. The memory made me feel even worse. "Adrian, I don't think I should."

He began pulling on flippers. "Then I'll go in," he said gruffly. "If you're going to work, I won't be long. You'll need *someone* to talk to."

Studying his disappointment, I decided abruptly that what he asked of me wasn't very much, really. He *had* helped me. And he was sympathetic and friendly, which seemed a rare commodity at Finisterre.

"Oh, come on!" I said. "Now that I'm here, I might as well!"

I pulled on the flippers, altering the strap to

fit feet that were smaller than the owner's. Picking up the tube and mask, I walked down into the water to put them on.

"Whose flippers are they?" I found him staring at me when I looked back.

"I bought them for Jane to use. Her feet are bigger than yours, aren't they? I'll adjust the straps if they're too tight."

"I already have." I tried the adhesion of the mask, and, satisfied, walked in and started swimming, presently hearing him following behind with long, strong strokes. Lending me Jane's flippers was adding insult to injury. Jane would probably rub them with poison ivy.

"Where did you learn to do that?" he demanded breathlessly, catching up.

"I told you. We had a house on the beach near Santa Monica."

"Now I know how you swam back against the beginning of the ebb," he said grimly. "Okay. Come down and take a look at my private world. Follow me, and stop when I do. Okay?"

He rolled and speared down. I followed him down into a world I'd loved ever since my father first taught me to snorkel when I was a child. The sun on the water gleamed above as we swam into a twilight world of greenish yellow, where tall red-brown kelp writhed and danced. Tiny fish ahead, suspended motionless in the clear water, parted to let us through. He motioned me deeper and began to show me things.

A green-and-red moray came partly from its

hole to stare at us with beady eyes as Adrian parted the kelp in exactly the right place. They treated each other with the calm contempt of old friends, the moray pretending not to notice Adrian as it watched me suspiciously. In a cavern under the cliff a fish that must have weighed eighty pounds, a big slow old thing with the biggest mouth I'd ever seen, stared back at us as the moray had done, without fear or emotion.

Adrian caught a lobster in a crevice, showed it to me, and put it back. Becoming more and more interested, I began to signal by touching his shoulder when I saw something he apparently hadn't noticed. Flowerlike sea anemones waving petals colored like sunflowers, chrysanthemums, gerberas. Once it was *I* who deliberately disturbed a sea anemone and made it shorten its stem and draw in its tentacles to show him the protective circular muscle closing up the whole creature as though in a leather bag.

He found a sea horse and showed it to me. I discovered a patch of kelp with leaves like yellow spaghetti. We came up to replenish the air supply in our masks, and he gestured down again, his eyes pleading. I weakened and smiled, and he was rolling, diving again. Turning over, I was surprised to find Jane Buchan standing on the beach staring at us, a towel trailing forgotten from her hand. I had forgotten Jane; so had Adrian, I was sure.

I followed his dark form down through the clear water. The kelp beds grew deeper, taller.

A solid rock wall loomed above us; then we were threading our way between clumps of kelp. It grew darker ahead. Adrian was swimming up. I followed, aware of a nervousness I couldn't understand. A rock thrust up ahead, shaped like a cathedral spire. He pointed at it and vanished, swimming around it. Kelp that grew tall ahead was parted as though by some current, forming a tunnel of kelp into which he was swimming now. It was dark in there, darker than I expected. My nervousness became fright as darkness, thickening, closed in about me. I swam faster, as he was swimming, eager to be through this weird place with the thick brown leaves waving mysteriously in the current, touching my body with slimy fingers.

The kelp was gone suddenly, but there was no relief from the darkness or the sense of confinement that was frightening me. And suddenly, as my hand touched stone, I realized the cause of my growing terror. We had been entering a natural tunnel, a blow hole through which the tide breathed, that led into the bowels of the cliff. A tunnel masked by the tall kelp, camouflaged, hidden. *We were already in it!* Entering a world of complete darkness. To me a world of terror! There was no room to turn back, unless you were a contortionist. I wanted to scream and turn back, but I could not.

Light flooded back to me suddenly, showing me the narrow tunnel in which I was trapped. *He had a flashlight.* The light replaced my terror with anger. To bring it he must have intended to lead me unsuspecting into this horrible tunnel beneath the sea. His treachery was premeditated.

The tunnel took all my attention then. There was barely room to flutter hands and flippers, and in my fright I was using up the air in my mask too quickly.

Suddenly then the tunnel began widening, and Adrian started angling up. I swam with him, staying in the light behind him. Water splashed before my mask. We had surfaced in this dark, terrifying place. Adrian was swimming on the surface. I watched him pull himself up out of the water. He sat waiting for me, legs dangling, calmly dragging off his mask.

The flashlight guided me to where he waited, and he caught my wrist and helped me up beside him. I dragged off my mask, grateful to breathe fresh, cool air, but more angry than I'd ever been in my life.

"I told you I didn't want to dive into your caves!" I told him furiously.

"I'm sorry!" His triumph faded as he studied my expression. "Are you angry with me? You were in no danger, and I thought you'd like it."

"Suppose I'd panicked when I discovered what you were doing to me? Suppose I'd tried to turn back and got *stuck*?"

"You're too good at underwater swimming to do that," he said. "I knew you would realize as well as I did we *had* to swim through into here to get the air to return to the surface. You did realize these things, didn't you, Samantha?"

"Even if I did, that doesn't excuse you leading me in here the way you did, Adrian!" I told him furiously.

"So okay, I'm sorry," he said contritely. "I'll take you back right away. But first let me show you the beauty I found in here?"

"I don't like dark, confined places, subterranean caves, or caves beneath the sea, Adrian!" I told him coldly.

"Please? Just let me show you the roof?"

He moved the flashlight as he spoke, shining it across the water, letting the beam of light climb slowly from the surface of water, still agitated by our swimming, to the roof of this cave in which we sat with our legs dangling in the cold water. The wall of the cavern came to life with the light upon it, as though the tiny crystals of rock were diamonds reflecting the light in brilliant sparkles as it moved.

"Well, Samantha?"

"What is that?"

"Tiny sand crystals in the rock. Salt. There is some limestone in here, though most of it has washed away. The crystals in these substances reflect light. I'm proud of this place, and I think of it as mine, because I discovered it."

"It is beautiful," I admitted sulkily.

"Look over here. I wonder how long the sea took to shape this cave? A million years? Longer? I wonder who walked about in here before me? Indians? Prehistoric man?"

I watched with a growing fascination that made me forget my feeling of claustrophobia as I saw minute sparkling pinpoints of light, strata of different-colored rocks in the walls of a great cavern with a floor sloping back to the limit of the light's reach.

"You could hold a ball in here," he said in an awed voice. He got up, and not daring to be left behind, I followed him nervously across a level rock floor. "Can you imagine the effect chandeliers would have in here, Miss Walton? How an orchestra would resound within these walls? It could be a ballroom fit for an emperor!"

"Genghis Khan!" I muttered.

"You're making fun of me?" he said suspiciously.

"No, I meant it, Adrian!" His imagining was barbaric, it seemed to me. His flashlight had steadied, as though involuntarily, upon an opening high up in the back of the cavern. As it moved away, I asked almost guiltily, "What's in there?"

"Another, smaller cave. I never take anyone in. It isn't . . . beautiful like this one. I can't show it to you."

I smiled for the first time since I put on my mask. "One cave is more than enough for me, thank you. All I want is to go back topside into the sunshine again."

He had noticed my change of tone, for the light showed him my face briefly. "You're not angry anymore?" he asked hopefully.

"I'm *trying* not to be."

"Then you'll come here with me again?"

"*No!*" I said. You relent with someone like that, and you have it to do all over again. "Adrian, I understand how you feel about this place you've found. And it *is* beautiful, I admit, in an unearthly, an incredibly lonely way. But I find it too frightening to ever want to come here again. I'm being honest with you, Adrian. I have an unreasoning fear of confined, enclosed places like this. They *terrify* me. I must be claustrophobic. I feel I'm suffocating! Don't ask me to swim down here with you again."

"I'll take you back," he said glumly. "I'm sorry! I know some people react that way. I won't ask you to swim with me again."

He looked so dejected that I relented enough to say, "I'll *swim* with you again if you want me to, Adrian. But not down here. I was having a wonderful time until I found myself in the tunnel." I glanced around and shuddered. "The worst torture I could imagine for myself is to be trapped in a place like this, unable to get out!"

He had heard only the first part, I decided. His face lit up. "You *will* swim with me again?"

"*On the surface!*" I said grimly, pulling on my mask.

It was easier coming out, I had to admit. But my fear was still there. This time he made me hang on to one of his flippers and hold the light. When I saw how small the tunnel ahead really was, I felt I'd die of fright. I closed my eyes and gripped his flipper with all my strength.

I'd never been so pleased to see the blessed sunlight. When we swam back to the beach, Jane Buchan was gone.

7

I worked with a strangely subdued Adrian all afternoon. I was not much more communicative myself, for the realization that I had allowed him to lead me into an underwater cave had really shocked me. I had a hangover of reaction from what had happened, one that I knew from experience I wouldn't be rid of until I had a good night's sleep.

When we finally put away our gear and closed the library door just before dinner, he said unexpectedly, "It wasn't because I didn't want to show you the other cave, was it, Samantha? Jane often got furious because I wouldn't take her in there. Are you sure you're not just angry with me about that, the way she gets?"

I laughed. "Don't be silly, Adrian! I'm not Jane Buchan! I told you, I just can't take being in a confined space. When I make a telephone call at the drugstore, I have to leave the door of the booth open. I told you, I'm claustrophobic. I can't help it. It's a neurotic fear out of proportion to the stimulus. I've been told the cause, but there's nothing I can do about it. Except *avoid* going into any place like your cave!"

"You're sure it couldn't be like I said?"

I sighed. "No, it could not."

"I wouldn't frighten you like that intentionally. I never will again. I promise."

I smiled. "I don't intend to let you! I'm not blaming you, Adrian. You didn't know what you were doing to me. It's a terrible feeling. Like suffocation! But I felt perfectly safe with you until then. Like I told you, I'd swim with you again tomorrow—*but only on the surface.*"

I went up to my rooms to get ready for dinner, and he went downstairs.

In my room the sound of a car coming brought me rushing to my window with my heart thumping excitedly. But as I leaned out, looking eagerly for Paul, I saw that it was Pancho bringing Sara back in the pickup from the bus stop at the highway. I went back miserably to my preparation for dinner. Lucky Sara! She had probably spent a happy weekend with her boyfriend in Pescadero. Sara didn't know how lucky she was!

Jane Buchan served the dinner, but at least I could look forward to more pleasant company at meals tomorrow, now that Sara was back. Jane was icily polite when she had to speak to me about the meal. Whatever Mrs. Hacha said to her this morning had done some good, I thought. Only, as she took away the dishes and left me my coffee, she asked me bluntly if Adrian had taken me down to his secret cave.

"That was what he brought the snorkel and flippers for, wasn't it, Miss Walton?" she asked me sarcastically while I considered what to reply.

Her snorkel and flippers, as I supposed she thought of them.

"He showed me a cave," I said warily. "But . . ."

She stalked furiously out of the room with my dishes jangling before I could explain further. I took my time over the coffee, but she didn't come back. Now that the weekend was over, there seemed no point in calling Bel Air, so I went up to my room. Tomorrow, I decided, I'd phone Anne Amberg at the library. And I'd definitely call Harding, Harding, and Chadwick. I had a right to know what they were doing with my fiancé.

Meantime, what I needed most to recover from the worst weekend I'd had in a long time was a good night's sleep.

I had been sleeping deeply and dreamlessly when something wakened me, something that had me sitting bolt upright in my bed in terror that prickled the hairs on the back of my neck. Some sound had wakened me, I was sure, though I had no memory of what it was. Something terrifying, for I was still trembling uncontrollably.

I stared around my room in fright, but nothing seemed there to scare me. My door was still securely closed. I'd been locking it nights ever since I learned I was the only person sleeping here on the third floor. I'd neglected to close the window I'd opened wide to look for Paul's coming when I saw Pancho bringing Sara home. The draperies were moving, billowing in a breeze coming up from the sea.

Perhaps the draperies blowing like that had swept something from the small table near the window? There had been a vase there, I remembered. Sara had emptied dead flowers from it before she went off for her weekend, saying Jane would put fresh roses in it for me in the morning. Jane hadn't, of course. But the vase had been there. The curtains blowing in the wind had knocked it off the table, but the thick carpet would prevent its breaking.

I sighed in relief, satisfied that I had found the source of the sound that had wakened me. The breeze coming in was cooler than I expected, but I did not bother to switch on my light and look for my robe and slippers. There would be no broken glass. My warm bed would seem even more attractive when I picked up the vase and closed the window.

It was a perfect night outside; the stars shone beautifully, but there was no moon. Steadying the draperies, I felt first to see if the vase was still on the table.

My fingers touched something cold, which I felt disbelievingly. *It was the vase!* I'd been wrong in my theory; no falling vase had wakened me. I glanced back nervously around my bedroom in a hasty search that only verified my first impression that nothing else was wrong. The sound, if there was one, must have come

from outside. Perhaps from somewhere in the
grounds below my window.

Parting the draperies, I peered out and
down. The house and gatekeeper-gardener Pancho's lodge were in darkness except for a faint
glow of light below me that I knew came from
the light in the ground-floor passage that
burned all night. And as I stared down, the
sound came again, shrill and distant and terrifying. *A woman's scream!*

Frozen in horror, I stared toward the sound
that had stopped abruptly, as though stifled or
cut off before it could reach its crescendo. It
had come from the beach or the sea beyond. I
was sure of it! Sometimes, though, my fear argued, gulls mewed like that in the night when
disturbed. I had heard them as a little girl lying in bed in the beach house, when my imagination had given the sound a more fearful
meaning that left me trembling in its wake,
with my head beneath the covers.

But I was not a little girl now. I was a
woman. And, my mind warned me, what I had
heard was too loud, too strong for mewing gulls
as far away as the beach. The sound that I had
heard was exactly what it had seemed. Down
there, either in the water or on the beach, a
woman had screamed in abject terror.

A woman in fear for her life!

And I alone had heard the sound. I was
remembering the strength of the ebb tide again
suddenly as I fought it to get back to the
beach. Was someone *drowning* down there?
Someone I might save? I ran to the bed and

found robe and slippers. Yesterday morning I had swum down there with Adrian, on the safe tide. The ebb would have begun around two P.M.

What time was it? I groped for my bedside clock and peered at the luminous hands. The ebb tide tonight would be an hour later. It was not yet two A.M. by my clock. There was still a good hour of flat tide before the ebb began. If someone was in trouble, it was not from the ebb tide.

I was running silently down the carpeted stairs almost without any conscious decision of mine. At the ground floor I stopped nervously. *Adrian, I should call Adrian.* But I had no idea which room was his, or where on the ground floor the staff bedrooms were. People drowned while those who might help them did things like that. Rescue in the sea had to be fast. I'd learned that watching the lifeguards on Santa Monica beach.

I went through the dining room and ran across the unkept lawns, too tense to feel the cold as I listened for the sound to come again. The night stayed silent, as though nature listened with me. There was no sound. Even the sea was placid and silent below the cliffs. I reached the top of the path breathlessly, and started down. I could see tiny waves making phosphorescent patterns on the sand, but there was no other movement down there. The sea was calm with the stillness of the top of the tide on a calm night with no wind.

I reached the sand and stopped to listen.

There was no sound whatever out there in the darkness. No movement. Nothing. I shivered, beginning to feel the cold standing here in deep shadow on the beach. And suddenly my impulsive decision in coming here began to seem foolish. I started walking along the beach staring at the dark waters and listening.

It could have been gulls I heard.

It could have been some other kind of bird in the grounds. Not on the beach at all. Night played strange tricks with sound.

I walked to the spot where Jane Buchan had sunbathed, watching with jealous eyes as I went swimming with Adrian. That had been a foolish impulse, I decided now. I had accepted too easily what Sara had said about Jane not being in love with Adrian. About her merely wanting him because he was the only man available at Finisterre. And I had been grateful to Adrian Hacha for his sympathy and help. But I was not interested in Adrian—I was in love with Paul. And Sara could be wrong. How could you tell how another woman felt about a man?

I reached the end of the beach. Ahead I could see the dark shape of rocks, the cliff thrusting up.

"*Is anyone out there?*" I called to the sea.

I started back, stopping at intervals to appeal to the unresponding darkness. I would not make Jane Buchan jealous again, I decided, searching the sand for clothing, a towel, anything that might indicate someone had been foolish enough to swim in the darkness out there in the small hours of the morning.

"*Is anyone there?*"

I felt more foolish now, each time I called. *I* was the only person silly enough to be on this lonely beach in the cold at two in the morning. Even if Adrian and Jane swam in the nude here the way Sara said, they would have left towels, a robe, *something* lying on the sand for when they came out.

A wave wet my feet as it sneaked unsuspected out of the darkness. The water *was* warm enough for a night swim, but the air, this breeze coming in from the sea, was quite cold.

Swimmers would need to put something on when they came out of the water, but there was nothing here. I was wasting my time.

I warmed climbing back and running nervously across the lawns to the house. I had one bad moment when the door I had left unlocked refused to open, and I remembered Jane locking me out the morning before. My first thought when the door stuck was that they, Adrian and Jane that is, *had* been swimming down there but had got back first and locked me out. Pushing at the confounded door, I imagined myself shivering on the doorstep all night, unless I wakened the house by ringing the doorbell. And would I ever have some explaining to do then! Anxiety made me heave desperately.

The door gave so unexpectedly that I *fell* inside. I went nervously back to my room, and peeped into the bathroom and study before I could find courage to put out my light and crawl shivering beneath the covers.

I expected a smiling Sara to wake me this morning with an early-morning cup of coffee, but she did not. I slept late and had to rush to make it in time for breakfast after my adventurous night. But Sara was waiting when I walked into the dining room for breakfast, waiting to serve my favorite fruit juice and cereal.

She glanced toward the kitchen warily as I sat down, and bringing over my fruit juice, said in a low voice, I'm sorry I wasn't able to bring up your coffee this morning, Miss Walton, but Mrs. Hacha said I couldn't. Something happened last night. Mrs. Hacha said as there are only two of us to do the work now, the early-morning coffee has to go. It won't be for long, though. Mrs. Acton is sending down extra staff. A helper for Pancho, and some woman to replace Jane. Mrs. Hacha worked with her here before the Actons bought Finisterre. *She* sounds *gruesome*! She was a nurse here, like Mrs. Hacha."

I had been staring at her, feeling sick suddenly. "You said something happened last night. To ... to Jane Buchan?"

She glanced toward the kitchen and nodded. "They had a row last night, Mrs. Hacha and Jane. It's been brewing for a long time. I told you about Jane and Adrian. Mrs. Hacha doesn't like that. That's one thing, and Jane never pulled her weight, and she lets Mrs. Hacha see she hates her."

"What happened?" I asked, frowning.

"I had a fantastic weekend, so I went to bed early last night. They woke me up arguing in the kitchen, something about Adrian, and about Jane being insolent to you."

"She wasn't that bad, really," I said in Jane's defense, since Sara had put that to me as a question. "But Mrs. Hacha happened to hear what she said."

"Well, anyway, I went back to sleep. But this morning Mrs. Hacha called me earlier than usual. Half an hour earlier, and when I asked her why, she told me I'd have to manage the housework alone until someone came to take Jane's place, because Jane left on the late-night bus for Los Angeles, where she came from. She said she paid Jane off, and Jane isn't coming back. Then she told me about the other help coming here sometime today. Or tomorrow. She said after she fired Jane, Mrs. Acton happened to phone, and she arranged for the new staff."

I was aware of relief as I sighed. "Mrs. Acton always seems to phone late at night. I wonder why. Did Mrs. Hacha say? I mean, I've been expecting Mrs. Acton to call me, but she hasn't. And she didn't come here on the weekend as she promised."

"Maybe Mrs. Hacha will tell you why later, Miss Walton. It must be worrying for you."

"It is!"

"There's something else I haven't told you yet about last night," she said confidentially, lowering her voice. "You know we only have the pickup truck here for transport? It's old and noisy, and the garage is right next to my bedroom. I just can't help hearing it anytime Pancho has to start it and I'm in my bedroom. Well, it didn't wake me! After I went to sleep again, I didn't hear a thing."

"But you said you had a heavy weekend, you were tired."

"That old pickup, the way Pancho starts it, would wake the dead!" she said. "So I told Mrs. Hacha I didn't hear the pickup leave the garage, and the late bus gets to the intersection around three o'clock in the morning, so how did Jane get to the bus?"

I stared at her, frightened again suddenly as I remembered waking last night.

She smiled, slightly malicious. "Mrs. Hacha said I didn't hear the pickup leave *because Jane wasn't driven!* She said Jane was so impertinent when she told Jane she had to go, that she made Jane *walk* to the highway!"

"In the middle of the night like that?" I asked, shocked. "Carrying her own luggage?" I remembered my glimpse of black hair in a thicket and Mrs. Acton's chauffeur telling me about wild animals he'd seen in the forest. I shivered.

"Mrs. Hacha is a hard woman," Sara whispered, her eyes on the door. "It's *two miles* to the highway. It wouldn't worry Jane at first, not if she was in one of her tempers. But I'll bet once she cooled down in the dark in there among the trees, she ran all the way to the bus!"

"I know *I* would!" I said.

"*Me too!*" she echoed with feeling. "Look out!" She went off to the kitchen for my breakfast egg. Mrs. Hacha was coming in, her black eyes suspicious.

"Is everything to your satisfaction this morning, Miss Walton?" she asked.

"Perfect, thank you, Mrs. Hacha."

"Mrs. Acton phoned again last night. I told her you were anxious to hear from her, but she said it was too late to wake you. It was after two A.M. here, five A.M. where she was. She'd just flown in to La Guardia Airport, and she was very tired."

"Mrs. Acton is in *New York?*" I cried, startled.

"To meet Paul," she said calmly. "They're staying at the same hotel. Paul's employers sent him there because he did well on a disputed land claim in Arizona. She said to tell you Mr. Harding is more than pleased with him, and she said she'll tell Paul you're anxious and he's to call you today."

"Great!" I said. "But I haven't seen or heard from Paul in more than two weeks now, Mrs. Hacha, and nobody at Bel Air seems able to tell me where I can reach him. Can you give me the name of the hotel where they're staying?"

"So that you can call Paul yourself, Miss Walton?" she asked me coldly.

"Exactly."

"Mrs. Acton said Paul will call you today."

"She said Paul was coming here. She said before that that he would phone me. He didn't.

That isn't like Paul, Mrs. Hacha. I want to know why he hasn't called me, and I'm beginning to believe that only Paul is going to tell me that."

She studied my angry expression bleakly. "I can't tell you where they're staying, Miss Walton. Mrs. Acton didn't tell *me*. And as for Mrs. Acton promising to ask Paul to contact you when he did not, her son is an adult. She can't *make* him do things. Hasn't it occurred to you that *Paul* may not want to phone you? That he may not want to see you here at Finisterre or anywhere else? Men are like that, Miss Walton. Some tire quickly of a pretty face."

"You don't know Paul, Mrs. Hacha!" I told her angrily.

"I have a son of my own, Miss Walton," she said. "Which reminds me—Adrian is ill. He won't be working with you today. I've given him sedation."

"You've given him sedation?" Even close to tears, as she had brought me with her vindictive remark about Paul, that had puzzled me.

"I am a fully qualified nurse, Miss Walton," she reminded me coldly.

I watched her go back toward the kitchen while I held back tears at the thought of Paul rejecting me the moment I was out of sight. I hadn't pursued him. Not ever. It was he who had pursued me. It was Paul who fell in love first, not me. Paul who first suggested marriage.

But I had learned to love him in the same way he loved me now, deeply and tenderly, and nobody could tell me I was just a pretty face to him, one he would exchange at the first chance.

That idea was as incredible as that *I* would be likely to want anyone else, ever.

My egg and my coffee forgotten, I fled, holding back tears. As Sara brought the rest of my breakfast from the kitchen, she stared at me in surprise. The sympathy in her eyes completed my collapse.

"Don't you *want* your breakfast, Miss Walton?"

I could only shake my head, my lips compressed to contain my sobs as the tears began to flow. I fled upstairs, leaving poor Sara staring after me. Behind my locked door I cried myself out, about the way I had when in my early teens my mother and father were quarreling before they made it unbearable for each other and parted. There was relief in it, I knew from experience. And I supposed, as I began to calm at last, that these were also tears of self-pity, as they had been then.

I'd thought I would never again feel lost and alone when I fell in love with Paul Acton. But here was the same terrifying specter threatening me again.

I freshened up and forced myself to go back downstairs and phone Bel Air. If I could only speak to Paul, or even Vanessa, I knew I'd feel better. All I needed was a little reassurance. I couldn't believe that what was happening was any fault of Vanessa's. She had been aloof that first day, yes. But after that, I had seemed to win her affection. I believed she liked me.

Hadn't everything she said or did since been designed to help me?

But if I believed Vanessa had grown to like and accept me, then I must believe what Mrs. Hacha said about Vanessa asking Paul to contact me. And if I believed that, it was *Paul* who didn't want to phone me or see me.

That I could never believe! Not unless I heard it from Paul himself.

It took a long time for the call to get through, and the girl at the exchange to answer politely, "I'm sorry, madam, but your number is not answering."

"Will you try again, please? I insisted. It's awfully important. It's a big house, and there has to be someone there."

Like life-or-death important, almost, miss. This time she was quicker. "I'm sorry, madam. Your number is still not answering. I'm afraid there's nobody there."

"Thank you."

I put the phone down. *Nobody there?* But that was impossible. The house of a wealthy family like the Actons had servants, people who lived there all the time to keep the house functioning when the owners were away. You just couldn't go away and leave a house like that empty. Not unless you sent away the servants and put the house in mothballs and left some security service to keep an eye on it. And you only did that if you, the family, intended going off to some distant place, like New York, for six months or even a year.

I put the phone down and climbed the stairs

to the library and tried to work. Halfway
through the morning, an anxious Sara brought
me coffee that I couldn't drink. I couldn't bring
myself to tell her my troubles, so she went
away sympathetic but still curious. I gave up
after that. Not knowing what to do, I went out
into the grounds, wandering about alone, trying to think, to understand why Paul, my Paul,
didn't come driving in through the great iron
gates of Finisterre to comfort and reassure me.
I found I had walked to the path down to the
beach and was just standing there staring
down.

I shuddered as I remembered last night
again suddenly. Could the sound that had wakened me in fright that seemed to come from the
beach have been Jane Buchan and Adrian's
mother quarreling? Sara had said it was three
in the morning when the bus reached the intersection. It had been two when I heard the cry.
It could have been the same sounds I heard
that woke Sara—those two women quarreling.

But at two A.M.? For heaven's sake, *why* at
that time of night? Housekeepers just didn't
stay up till two A.M. to fire a girl like Jane for
impertinence. Puzzling, I started down the
path to the beach. Could Adrian and Jane have
met on one of their trysts, have been swimming
down here last night, but Adrian's mother
found out and waited up for them?

Sara said she heard Adrian's name mentioned.

I could see the length of the beach from
where I stood at the foot of the steps, and there

was nothing lying anywhere. No towel. Nothing. There had been nobody swimming down here last night to cry out for help. I was turning to climb back to the house again when I noticed the shed. Hadn't someone told me it was used for dressing? That was the one likely place where someone night-swimming might leave their towel or their robe that I hadn't thought of last night when searching.

I had to walk around the steps to get to where it stood at the back of the beach under the steep slope that led up to the house. The door was unlocked, and opened when I pushed. A wooden shutter served as a window, but the shutter was closed and it was dark inside until I opened the door wide and let in the sun. There was no shower, just a bench for people to sit on, and at the back of the shed a cupboard for clothes.

If anything had been left here, I expected it to be left on the bench, carelessly. But it might be in the cupboard. I couldn't leave without checking.

Crossing the rough wooden floor, I stopped to peer down. Something had gleamed in the light from the door, something gold. I bent to pick it up and stare down at it, a plain gold cross on a broken chain. I had seen it before somewhere. Somewhere? *Of course*! Jane Buchan wore a gold cross on a chain like this one.

I carried it to the door and examined it curiously, turning it over. There was in inscription on the back, I saw. "To Jane with love from A. Summer of '76."

I stared at it, wondering. Had Adrian given her that last summer? She must have lost it here when the chain broke. She must have changed in here yesterday morning. She had been gone when I came from the cave with Adrian. She could have lost it then. I had turned to walk back to the cupboard when Adrian's voice called to me from the steps.

"What are you doing in there, Samantha? You're not going swimming alone, are you?"

"I'm not going swimming at all," I called back. "I thought you were sick. Your mother told me she had to give you sedation last night, and that you wouldn't be working today. I wasn't working well, so I walked down here to clear my head. I looked into the dressing shed and found this." Coming back to the door, I dangled it by the chain, showing him the cross.

"That's *Jane's!*" he said, staring at it.

"Yes, I know. I've seen her wearing it. She must have dropped it in here yesterday morning. She was gone before we left the water."

"Yes, of course," he said. "*Yesterday* morning."

"I was just going to look in the cupboard to see if she's left anything else behind. Your mother did tell you she's left Finisterre, didn't she?"

"Yes, she did," he said shortly. "But you needn't look in the cupboard. There's nothing in there. I woke up with a head full of cotton from the tablets my mother gave me last night.

The best cure I know for that is a swim, so I changed in there, and the cupboard was bare when I left my pajamas and robe in there. I didn't notice the cross. Where did you find it?"

I came down the steps and gave it to him. "On the floor. Is the A for Adrian?"

"Yes," he admitted. "I gave it to Jane last summer. Will you do something for me, Samantha? Don't tell my mother you found it, or about the inscription." He hesitated. "I'd like to . . . to be the one who returns it to Jane. Do you mind?"

I smiled affectionately. "Of course not, Adrian. Are you coming back to the house?"

He shook his head, still holding the cross in his hand. "No, I think I'll stay here, walk awhile. I'll come back to work after lunch."

"I heard at breakfast that Jane had gone," I said awkwardly. "I'm sorry your mother blamed her for being rude to me. I didn't mind what she said, or complain about it. It was just that your mother happened to hear."

"Yes, I know that," he said. "But there were other things. Things you don't know about, Samantha. What happened to Jane was not of your doing. My mother hated her."

He turned away from me and began to walk slowly away along the beach with the broken chain dangling from the hand that held the cross.

Poor Adrian, I thought with compassion, for I had seen tears in his eyes. But I had my own private sorrow. I began to climb the steps with all my own problems rushing back. I glanced up as I reached the top of the path and stopped abruptly, staring up. I had seen that same vagrant gleam of light up there under the eaves of Finisterre. And, yes, it was coming from the third window on the right, as Mrs. Hacha said. And the draperies were slightly apart. I could see that more clearly from up here. Only, as I stared up at the window, the gleam of sunlight on glass vanished abruptly, and momentarily I thought I saw a dark shape move.

But my problems had returned to torment me, and whatever it was up there, sunlight on window glass or whatever, it was gone.

I began to walk back to the house.

8

I had worked with a strangely subdued Adrian all day. He worked listlessly and without interest, his old zest for helping me completely gone. I blamed Jane Buchan's hasty departure from Finisterre for his aberration today, and tried to draw him out about his feeling for Jane, hoping that he might relieve some of his tensions that way. But the very mention of her name made him clam up and withdraw deeper into the mood of depression that possessed him. He became paler and more depressed as the day wore on, and by late afternoon looked positively ill. When I told him he should go to his room and rest, he agreed gratefully.

I stopped work soon afterward myself, remembering my own problem. I couldn't go on like this, waiting for Paul or Vanessa to call me or to come to Finisterre. The next time Vanessa phoned, it was just as likely to be from London, or Berlin, or some even more distant place.

Working, I decided on two moves I'd make.

First I would call Harding, Harding, and Chadwick's Los Angeles office, no matter how difficult Mrs. Hacha said it was to call there long distance from Finisterre. I'd demand to know *where* my fiancé was staying in New York. And once I found that out, I'd call Paul person-to-person at his hotel.

And tonight I would call Anne at the Stanford library. We'd been friends too long to drift apart just because Anne had left her Palo Alto apartment next to mine and I was stuck here at Finisterre. It would be a comfort just talking to Anne. She was a down-to-earth girl with lots of common sense. Anne would know what I should do to find Paul, if I could not find out anything from Harding, Harding, and Chadwick.

Only, as I planned this, I remembered suddenly that Anne didn't know where I was. She was away from her apartment the day I made my hasty decision to go to Finisterre as Vanessa wished. A decision I was regretting more with each passing day.

Back in the sanctuary of my room, I stared out of the window, working on my problems. The ebb tide was running out to sea like a millrace. Someone had built a fire of driftwood in the corner of the beach near the dressing shed. Pancho, I supposed disinterestedly, keeping the beach tidy. But as I stared down, the man who had lit the fire came out of the dressing shed, and it wasn't the Mexican gardener—it was Adrian Hacha. Adrian carried what looked like a bundle of old clothes in his arms, and as I

watched, he threw them on the leaping flames
from the dry wood. The pungent smell of burning rags drifted up on thickening smoke. Something in the bundle blazed high as it caught
alight, burning with the intensity of some flam-
mable nylons.

Then the fire began to smoke. I watched,
only partly understanding. Adrian hadn't gone
to his room to forget his troubles, he had gone
down to the beach instead. But perhaps burning old forgotten clothing from the dressing
shed was some chore his mother had given him.
I turned away, losing interest. It was time to
start trying if I wanted to call Harding,
Harding, and Chadwick.

I heard Mrs. Hacha's voice giving Sara in-
structions about dinner as I came downstairs. I
closed the door of the living room quietly, shut-
ting out Mrs. Hacha's harsh voice. Paul had
written the office phone number on a page torn
from his notebook at the airport, I remembered
nostalgically as I looked at it. The memory
made me want to cry. Everything had seemed
so uncomplicated for us that evening. Our future had never seemed brighter.

I made the call, speaking quietly, and
waited. Ten minutes, fifteen, twenty. It was
eerie in the living room with its closed draperies, and it kept growing darker and darker.

There was a telephone in the kitchen, another in Mrs. Hatcha's office, another in the library. Would the call register on them all?
Would the housekeeper pick up a phone if she
heard the call, and listen in?

I grabbed for the phone as it began to burr, taking me by surprise, even though I was waiting for it.

A woman's pleasant voice asked, "Can I help you?"

I kept my voice down. "I'm trying to contact Paul Acton?"

"We seem to have a bad connection; will you speak louder, please?"

"I'm trying to find out how I can contact Paul Acton."

"Mr. Acton is away on business. Who *is* that speaking, please?"

"This is Samantha Walton, Paul's fiancée," I said. "It's most urgent that I contact Paul or his mother quickly. They're staying in New York. Can you give me the name of their hotel, please? Or better still, the hotel phone number?"

Her voice changed, became hostile suddenly, as though at the mention of my name. "Mr. Acton has been working in Arizona with Mr. Chadwick, one of our senior partners. They're driving home by way of the ranch that was the subject of the litigation, and they intend to stay there overnight."

"Then if you will give me the phone number of the ranch, I can call Paul *there!*" Momentarily, at the thought of that, I was delighted. Just to hear Paul's voice, to speak to him again . . .

"I'm sorry," her voice said coldly, "But we are not allowed to divulge information like that about our clients. And I'm not sure that Mr.

Acton would want to hear from *you*, Miss Walton. Not after the shabby way you treated him!"

"What did you say?" I gasped." I'm not sure I understand."

"Here we sympathize with Mr. Acton—he's a fine young man!" she said. This time I couldn't doubt her hostility—she cut me off.

I was frightened now, really frightened. Things were happening that were beyond my understanding. I *needed* a friend. *I needed Anne!* I reached for the phone again.

The lights in the big room came on abruptly. Mrs. Hacha's voice said harshly from the doorway: "What are you sitting in here in the dark for, you foolish girl?"

I jumped guiltily. "I'm trying to call a girlfriend of mine in Palo Alto. We worked together and lived in adjoining apartments."

"Really?" she said. "Long-distance calls cost money!" She said it as indignantly as though *she* had to pay for them.

"I make a note of my calls, and *I* intend to pay for them, Mrs. Hacha."

She sniffed disdainfully. "Your dinner will be ready on time. See that you are, Miss Walton!" She went out and closed the door. I listened to her walk briskly back to the kitchen before I called the Stanford library number. A bored, familiar voice answered, as I had myself many, many times.

"Stanford library, yes?"

A voice I knew well. But not Anne's voice. I smiled nevertheless.

"Jan Carter?"

"Yes. Who is that?"

"Samantha Walton."

"*Sam*? We all thought you eloped with that fantastic blond guy you were dating. What's-his-name."

"Paul Acton? We *are* engaged. Jan, it's important that I speak to Anne. Please?"

"You mean Anne Amberg? Don't you know Anne doesn't work here anymore?"

"What?" I cried in dismay.

"Oh, she's coming back for the next term," she said reassuringly. "But some realtor firm took over the apartment house where Anne lived. They paid her plenty to transfer the lease, and guaranteed to find her another apartment elsewhere. Don't ask me why. But with what they gave her, Anne doesn't have to work in the library this vacation. She went off someplace to have a vacation herself on the money. She didn't say where. Lucky Anne!" She broke off abruptly. "Hey! Didn't *you* live in the same apartment house? Did they buy you off too? I'll bet that's why you disappeared without even saying good-bye. How lucky can girls get?"

"I've been staying at my fiancé's mother's beach house," I said in denial. "I didn't even know this was happening!"

"Then you'd better find out about it pretty quick, Sam," she said seriously. "Or *you* just might find yourself without an apartment. And you'd have to be an heiress to pay the new rent in that building, they tell me. Say, if I were you I'd call the apartment right away!"

"I mean to!" I said grimly. I hung up quickly, glanced at the door, and dialed again. After a wait, an unfamiliar woman's voice answered.

"Mrs. Canning here. Can I help you?"

"A friend just informed me the new management has been buying the leases of the previous tenants, and that most of them have gone."

"This is true. Why do you ask, Miss . . . ?"

"Walton, Samantha Walton. I've leased apartment twenty-one for the last three years. I'm on vacation, and this is the first I've heard. Can you tell me what is happening about it?"

"I'll check," she said. "Hold the line, Miss Walton."

I waited uneasily for her voice to return. "Your lease expired more than two weeks ago, Miss Walton," she said. "You neglected to renew the lease or contact us in any way. A new tenant moved into twenty-one."

I stared at the phone disbelievingly. "You can't *do* that! I've renewed the lease each year. The former management, the Methodists, always held the same apartments for students. They *knew* I needed it for another year!"

"You should read your leases more carefully, Miss Walton," she said, not without sympathy. "You were given fourteen days following the expiration of the lease to renew. You failed to do this. That renewal period ended three days ago. However, we are prepared to give you favored treatment as a former tenant, if we can. I suggest you see us quickly, though. Apartments in Palo Alto are hard to get."

As though I didn't know that! "Who do I ask for?" I asked her miserably. "For you, Miss Canning?"

"You don't come *here*, Miss Walton," she said in an amused voice. "I'm afraid you'll have to go to Los Angeles. Our head office is on the corner of Lincoln and Jessop. Ask for Mr. Gleeson and tell him I sent you. I should warn you, though, you'll find the rents much higher now. Acton has made fantastic improvements to the apartments, which were very ordinary."

I was staring at the phone suddenly. "You said *Acton*?"

"Why, yes, of course," she said. "Acton Realtors are the new owners."

I put the phone down slowly, disbelievingly. Acton Realtors, Paul had told me, belonged to Vanessa Acton. The more I thought about that, the more frightened I became.

For it seemed to me that in the inexplicable web of my problems a pattern of duplicity was emerging clearly for the first time.

Suppose Vanessa hadn't told Paul I was at Finisterre?

Like the jigsaw puzzles I'd been given when I was a little girl, the pieces that had puzzled me most were falling unexpectedly into place.

I remembered Vanessa winning my confidence at the hotel, discovering that my parents had divorced and remarried. Discovering that I was all alone. It was Vanessa who had arranged for Paul to be offered the job with her attorneys in distant Los Angeles. It was Vanessa who, when he accepted the job, con-

vinced Paul that going even farther away, to
Phoenix, Arizona, must lead to a junior partnership.

I had been wondering why Paul didn't come
to Finisterre, or phone me here, because this
sort of neglect just wasn't like Paul. But I
hadn't been given the chance to tell Paul that I
was coming here. Vanessa had said *she* would
do that, and by the time I began to worry, Paul
was gone. My promise to Vanessa not to tell
Paul had been a part of her wonderful scheme
to give me a holiday vacation by the sea, yet at
the same time enable me to earn the money I
had to have for rent of the apartment in Palo
Alto when my postgraduate studies began with
the next semester. An apartment that now belonged to Vanessa's Acton Realtors.

I began to understand the cold dislike in the
voice of the woman at Harding, Harding, and
Chadwick's office now. *She thought I'd walked
out on Paul!* And Paul—what must Paul be
thinking? Where would he have tried to find
me? Certainly not here at Finisterre! Even at
the library they hadn't known I was here until
I told Jan Carter just now. If he found Anne,
Anne couldn't help him. Vanessa Acton's chauffeur had whisked me away before I could tell
Anne. Even Mrs. Pettit, our kindly apartment
supervisor, couldn't help Paul. Mrs. Pettit had
been fired.

I'd be wasting my time and money if I flew
to Los Angeles to ask for a new lease. Vanessa
didn't want *me* anywhere where Paul could
find me!

I had discovered my danger now. But this was only part of the jigsaw. There had to be more than this, *much more*, I was realizing with growing fear, sitting alone in the darkness of the great living room of Finisterre.

What had Vanessa told Paul about me? *How* had she explained what must have seemed to Paul my inexplicable disappearance? I thought of the dislike in the voice of the woman from his office.

"I'm not sure Mr. Acton would want to hear from *you*," she had told me bluntly. "Not after the shabby way you treated him!"

Had Vanessa told Paul I didn't want to go through with our wedding? Paul's first impulse, I knew, would be to find me, if she told him that. As I felt about Paul, so Paul felt about me. Neither of us would accept rejection at second hand. Paul would demand to hear that from me, not from Vanessa.

I got up quickly. I must escape from this horrible Finisterre on its lonely cliff beside the sea, where Vanessa Acton had trapped me. I must escape and find Paul. *Now!* Only, as I hurried to the door, I heard a car coming in through the gates. Its lights reflected upon the window in the darkness, showing in grim silhouette the iron bars the draperies concealed.

Someone from the outside world was coming to Finisterre! I ran to the living-room door and tore it open.

"Is something the matter, Miss Walton?" a sarcastic voice asked. Mrs. Hacha, coming unnoticed from her kitchen, was studying me where I poised in the doorway. "You've been acting strangely tonight, haven't you? Sitting in there in the dark making telephone calls. And now I find you standing in the doorway staring at Sara opening the front door. Are you expecting someone?"

"I heard a car come in. I thought Paul, or perhaps Vanessa . . . ?"

She shook her head, holding her malicious smile that tonight hinted at some secret triumph. "The car is bringing new staff members Mrs. Acton has sent me. Reliable people I know I can trust to carry out even unpleasant tasks. I know, because I've worked with them here before."

"Mrs. Hacha is expecting you," Sara's voice said with nervous politeness at the door.

I turned quickly to look at the newcomers, but found no hope there. A woman as tall and strong-looking as Mrs. Hacha had brushed past Sara and was walking toward us. She had gray hair and a hard, masculine face. The man followed heavily behind her, two traveling bags held carelessly in one large hand, a brutish-faced man whose eyes crawled over my flesh with an unnatural interest as he noticed me standing in the doorway. The woman looked at me coldly in passing, with expressionless blue eyes. She raised her eyebrows in silent interrogation as she looked at Mrs. Hacha.

"Miss Walton is our *only* guest," Mrs. Hacha said, as though in explanation of me. "If you and Karl will follow me, Ingrid, I'll show you to your rooms."

"It's been a long time, Catherine," the woman said. The man looked at me again and followed the woman silently. I felt myself shiver, though the night was warm.

Why had Vanessa thought it necessary to send people like these to Finisterre? Or had that been Catherine Hacha's idea? My heart thumped sickly as I watched them follow the housekeeper toward the kitchen. In imagination I saw myself incarcerated forever in Finisterre, guarded by the two horrible people who had stared at me in passing. Perhaps they meant to lock me in one of those grim cells on the top floor where once the violent mental patients had been kept in maximum security, guarded by these very people.

"*Miss Walton!*"

I had forgotten the maid, but Sara was whispering my name, her hand on my arm persuading me to move back into the shadows of the living room with her.

"Who are those people, Miss Walton?" she whispered. "They're scary, aren't they? I'm going to lock my door tonight!"

"Mrs. Hacha said they're new staff Mrs. Acton hired."

"*Those two?* To take the place of Jane Buchan? That woman doesn't look like any lady's maid to me! And that man! *Miss Walton, I'm scared!*"

She wasn't the only one! I nodded. At the moment, I could think of only one thing, *escape!* Like Jane Buchan, I was going to walk to the highway through the woods. I couldn't take much with me. Yet, all my worldly possessions were up there in my bedroom. Vanessa had arranged that too! Bring all your things, dear Samantha! Leave no trace of yourself behind in the apartment for Paul to find. Leave no trace that he can follow!

"Miss Walton, there's something else," Sara whispered, with a quick glance down the passage. "I take her afternoon coffee to her office. This afternoon she was talking to someone on the phone. A man. He asked for Mrs. Acton, but she said Mrs. Acton wasn't here. He must've argued about that, because she said she was sure Mrs. Acton was not coming to Finisterre."

"So what?" I said curtly, only half-understanding. In flight, I couldn't carry my gear two miles through the forest, I was thinking. Nor could I wait until those horrible people organized by Catherine Hacha as my guards made escape impossible.

"She lied," Sara muttered. "That's what. She told me earlier to prepare Mrs. Acton's rooms because she was coming here tonight. Mrs. Acton was in the car with these people. I just saw her. She went into Mrs. Hacha's office by the side door."

"Vanessa is *here*?" I stared at her, shocked, with my terror growing. Vanessa, the woman, Ingrid, and the man—were these the last parts of the jigsaw?

"Sara!" Mrs. Hacha's voice called impatiently.

"She's missed me! I'll have to go," Sara

gasped. "But why did she lie about that to Paul?"

"To Paul?" I stared at her disbelievingly. "You mean Paul Acton? My fiancé?"

"I'm almost sure it was Paul, Miss Walton. When she stayed here to fix your room, she had me call him for her twice. The voice seemed the same."

I caught her arm as she moved to go. "Where was Paul calling *from*?"

"I don't know. I couldn't let her see I was listening. I had to pour her coffee and leave. But somewhere not far away, I thought."

"Is there some way I could find out?" If Paul was close, even in San Francisco or Palo Alto . . .

"*Sara!*" Mrs. Hacha's voice called, suspicious and angry now.

She gasped and pulled away from my hand in fright. "I *could* call Dad! He might be able to find out."

I remembered her telling me her father was a police officer in Pescadero. Maybe he *could* trace the call. But that took time. "No!" I called after her, but doubted that she heard.

I stood there shaking. If I'd only been in the library, I might have picked up the phone, and I would've recognized Paul's voice! But it must have happened while I was at the window of my room watching Adrian burn old clothes! I couldn't expect Paul to phone again. He'd been told Vanessa wasn't here. My fear warned me to go quickly *now*. In my room I crammed a few things hastily into an overnight bag, dragged on jeans and sneakers for my walk through the woods, and took what money of my own I had. A few dollars only. I'd received none for my work here; Vanessa had made sure of that too. With money, I might escape. I left the light on in my bedroom and crept downstairs, trembling. I could hear voices in the kitchen. A man's deep voice, Sara answering nervously.

The dining room had a side door that opened onto the gravel drive. The dining-room door was open, and beyond it I could see the side door that seemed to lead to safety.

Beyond the dining-room door that I stared at, vacillating, the living-room door opened abruptly, scaring me stiff. Ingrid was coming out! Beyond her, Catherine Hacha sat at a table with a glass of sherry in her hand, giving Ingrid orders before she closed the door.

I froze in terror, peering wide-eyed between the banisters. I was sure Catherine Hacha must see me where I crouched on the stairs trying to make myself smaller. But she was not alone in the living room, I saw now. Someone else was sharing that table and the sherry. A woman who held the gleaming crystal glass of sherry gracefully by slim fingers with red-painted nails. I could see the other woman's hand and wrist and part of her forearm. She wore a platinum bangle studded with diamonds that . . .

I stared at the bangle, shocked. Wanting to run for that tempting open door but afraid to try. *Vanessa*! Her hand and arm disappeared as she raised the glass to sip sherry.

Ingrid said, "Of course, at once, Catherine." To my horror, she came striding toward the stairs. I closed my eyes like a frightened rabbit and crouched, waiting to be discovered, while the pounding of my heart drowned the sound of Ingrid's feet in the deep carpet, waiting to hear Ingrid's heavy tread upon the stairs, to feel her strong hands seize me and drag me back to face Vanessa and Mrs. Hacha.

Sickened by fear, I listened to those heavy footsteps reach the foot of the stairs and start to recede again, going on toward the kitchen as though I wasn't there. I opened my eyes, shaking, and let my held breath sigh out. Ingrid was just walking into the kitchen. She vanished without looking back.

Now! I must go now, before she came back or Mrs. Hacha came from the living room and saw me crossing the passage. I forced myself upright on trembling legs, courted disaster by almost stumbling and falling headlong down, so frightened was I. But my sneakers making no sound on the carpet, I crossed the passage to the open door.

One terrified glance showed me the huge shadow of Ingrid on the kitchen wall to spur me on across the dining room and outside into the darkness of night with fog rising from the sea. Fog, I hoped, would hide me in the forest if they found I was missing and came searching for me. I crept stealthily past the lighted living-room windows and hurried toward the gates. A light burned above the gate, another over the closed door of Pancho's stone cottage.

There was a light in the window there, and I heard Pancho cough as I reached the gates. I put down my overnight bag. How did the gate open? I pulled back a heavy bolt that squeaked protestingly even though I was being as quiet as I could.

I pushed the gate, but it refused to move! Perhaps it opened the other way. Inward? I pulled steadily, straining as my fear increased.

"You can't open it that way, senorita," a man's voice said triumphantly behind me. "There is also a lock. You need *this*."

Dangling keys on a ring from one fat hand, Pancho was grinning at me where he stood under the light above his door. A big man, overweight, his stomach bulged in a gray shirt and dirty white trousers.

With my heart starting a sick thumping, I held out my hand. "Give me the key, then."

He laughed, studying me. "Tell me why I should do that, senorita."

I remembered Jane Buchan suddenly. "You knew Jane Buchan, didn't you? Then you know that Mrs. Hacha fired her and made her walk to the highway. They've just done the same thing to me. So give me the key, or open the gate, Pancho. Or they may do the same to you."

"But you are wrong about the dark-haired one, senorita," he said. "If she left here, it was not through my gate. Therefore, she must still be here. And you are no maid, senorita, but a young woman who intended to take Senora Acton's son away from her, as the dark-haired one would have that fool Adrian."

"True—I'm Paul Acton's fiancée," I said, glancing back at the silent house. "And you will work for my husband one day, Pancho—*if* you are still here. Open the gate, and be quick! I have a long way to go!"

"But you are not going anyplace, señorita," he said. He raised his hand to touch something above his door on the inside. While I watched uncomprehendingly, I heard the shrill clamor of an alarm start ringing in the distant house.

He came after me at once, while I stood still, frozen in fright, and he was fast for such a fat man. But desperation moved me at the last moment to snatch up my overnight bag and run. His fingers caught the handle of the bag as I turned. I faced him, tugging at it, trying to take back my few possessions by force while he laughed triumphantly at my futile struggles, until I let go the bag and he staggered back foolishly to fall sprawling on the gravel drive. I was already running in the only direction I could take, toward the house and that jangling alarm.

I fled without the bag, running desperately as I saw light spill from the dining-room door I'd closed behind me, as the man Karl appeared there, staring out.

At sight of him, I swerved and ran toward the opposite side, where the great stone outer wall ran close to the house. The rooms on that side of Finisterre were little used. I ran in between wall and house, hearing the front door

open as I ran, and Mrs. Hacha's voice call to
Pancho.

Ahead, distantly, as I ran, I could see the
shape of trees. The cemetery was there, I
remembered, for I had avoided it when walking in the grounds.

Perhaps in there some tree that I could climb
stood close to the wall. I ran in terror toward
the trees and the shape of headstones.

9

I hid in a corner of the cemetery, staring back wide-eyed with terror toward the house. Back there, where tangled weeds and seeding grass covered what had once been neat gardens and lawns, flashlights were gleaming among the trees. It was as though everyone in Finisterre were out hunting me systematically. For they were working from the back of the house, spaced out, flashing lights and calling to one another in low voices.

The fog was thickening, but not quickly enough to hide me. And there was nowhere I could go, nowhere I could run to, it seemed to me as I crouched in terror, trying to think how I might escape from Finisterre and my pursuers.

"Look in the cemetery, Karl! Ingrid! Watch she doesn't double back!"

That was Adrian's mother, Catherine Hacha, organizing the hunt. I glanced around desperately. I had hoped to find some tree in the cemetery that I might climb to reach the top of the wall. There were none. That was an eventuality they must have foreseen when this horrible place was a lunatic asylum! If there had ever been trees growing close to the wall, they had long ago been removed.

Perhaps in the forest I might find one? Staring back, I saw a light moving in among the headstones near the entrance gate, with the bulky shadow of the man Karl looming behind its erratic beam of light.

I got up in terror and ran as stealthily as I could to the picket fence at the back of the cemetery. Once it had been painted white, but all that remained of paint now was a lessening of the color of wood that had long since weathered gray. I'd never tried to climb a picket fence before. If the rails the pickets were nailed to had been inside, it would have been easy. But there were only the perpendicular pickets on this side, with no grip for my feet from the ground to their blunt spearhead tops. I tried and fell, terrified. Karl was closer, swinging his light in half-circles, and just outside the cemetery fence I could see Ingrid, fifty yards closer than Karl, and searching the thickets as industriously.

I got up, shaking. The possibility of being caught in here by that man filled me with panic. Somehow I dragged myself to the top of the pickets, balancing precariously. Balancing, I found my foot had stuck! I had to turn sideways, groping for a foothold on the top rail with the other foot, both my hands gripping the picket tops while I tried to drag my foot upward and out to free it.

"*There she is!*" Ingrid cried in her mannish voice. "*Climbing the fence! Get her, Karl!*"

I gasped in horror as the light of her flashlight blinded me. I cried out and was falling, hearing Karl's triumphant shout as he came after me. The fall drove most of the breath from my body. I scrambled up and ran, aware that I had lost one sneaker, but too terrified to try to retrieve it or pull off the other shoe.

"She lost one shoe! It's stuck between the pickets! She can't get far!" Ingrid was coming, plowing through the underbrush outside the fence. Sobbing, I put my head down and ran in among the trees.

"Adrian! Watch the path!" I recognized his mother's voice beyond Ingrid. I glanced back. Karl was swearing, having as much trouble trying to climb that fence as I had. I hoped he'd fall and break a leg. The grounds ahead were narrowing, the walls closing in on me on either side. Terror sickened me as I saw that narrowing space ahead between high stone walls. There was no escape there. If I went on, I must be found and caught, even though I seemed to have drawn away from my pursuers, or they had slowed, sure of me now.

I stared around wildly. Veils of fog were spilling over the wall above the cliff, as on the night I came to Finisterre. The trees ended. Ahead, there was no place to hide, no room to run. The fog, when it came, must be too late to conceal me. Thought of never seeing Paul again gave me the strength to turn for the first time to face those dancing lights following me. For the first time since I had begun to run blindly from my pursuers, I began to reason.

I saw the gap in their advance at once.

I had almost missed it, it seemed to me. If they had moved quicker, drawing together as the stone walls did, I could not have escaped! But I could now, I saw, if I had the courage. On my left, Karl and Ingrid had drawn close together and were too far to the left. It was the same on the other side. Two lights there danced about, shining on the thinning trees, the thickets beneath. Mrs. Hacha and Pancho or Adrian must be there.

If I had the courage to hide and wait until they passed or drew level with me, I could outrun them, I was sure. If I could reach the gates, climb them, run into the forest . . .

With my heart thumping, I crouched beneath the nearest tree and took off my one shoe. I would run faster barefoot. The way of escape lay between the two women, Mrs. Hacha and Ingrid.

The tree I had chosen was as good as any here, where salt wind from the sea stunted them. The lights advanced slowly. They were walking, I saw, not running. I pressed against my tree, fighting a silly impulse to close my eyes.

Hugging my tree, I watched them come. The lights came closer, drew level. I dared not run yet. Karl had lagged behind Ingrid. He might head me off, if he was a fast runner. He . . .

"There's her other shoe! Look out, there she is behind the tree!" Ingrid's harsh voice called.

My tree and I were bathed in blinding light. I was running, hearing their voices behind rise excitedly as they gave chase. Worse, as I began to run, I saw the flashlight on my left dancing about as someone running very fast drew level with me and began to forge ahead. I gasped in terror. *Karl!* Karl was going to head me off, just as I had feared!

I spurted, holding him, but he was a good twenty yards ahead on my left, and he was running as fast as I was, dodging between the trees with astonishing agility for such a big man. And suddenly I realized that, slowly, stealthily, his path was converging with mine.

I began to edge right, as he was doing, moving closer to the wall, the cliff, the sea.

"Catch her, Karl, she's got no place to go!" a woman's voice urged behind me.

My pumping lungs hurt, and a pain began to burn in my side. I was drawing away from the pursuers behind me, but not from Karl. There he was, ahead, moving in like a shepherd dog herding some silly runaway sheep, driving me ever closer to the wall. Then I remembered the path down to the beach. There was the break in the wall above sheer cliff just ahead, the beginning of the first steps down.

To my horror, a new light flashed suddenly ahead, directly in front of me a hundred yards or so beyond the path to the beach. Someone was there, waiting for me! I had no choice now. It was the beach, or capture. And if they caught me, what then? Did Vanessa intend to have them hide me away, a prisoner in one of those horrible upstairs rooms? I remembered the tide down there, ebbing, running like a mill-race! But that was hours ago. The tide must be nearing changing. I had lost count of time. I wondered if they had too.

The path was ahead, and Karl had run past it. The new light was coming fast. I chose the beach. That must be Adrian who had closed the door of the trap upon me by appearing unexpectedly ahead, I decided hopelessly. Even *Adrian* had turned against me now.

I started down on shaking legs; momentarily, the new flashlight shone full upon me as I went down on unsteady legs weakened by effort and not yet adjusting to such things as steps. Then the light went out.

"She went down!" Karl's thick voice called exultantly.

"Don't let her sneak back!" Catherine Hacha called breathlessly.

If he replied, I didn't hear. It would have taken all my concentration to find the steps in the darkness and the fog, even if my legs hadn't been converted to jelly by the descent. The fog caught up with me. It writhed, enveloping me with cold dampness. The sea seemed quieter. Perhaps the tide was already changing. But hope faded as I came closer. A maelstrom of water was boiling out there over the reefs. I staggered in sand softer than I expected, and glanced back in terror, listening. If they were coming, they made no sound, were using no lights. Why?

Perhaps they were closer than I thought. That

started me running again along the hard wet sand at the water's edge. And as I ran, in my mind I began to see a new pattern of terror emerging. I had been *driven* to the beach. Deliberately. The gap between the searchers, Karl falling back. The waiting light beyond the path to the beach designed to turn me toward the only way of escape left—the sea. The sea on an ebb tide that Vanessa was sure would drown me. All this had been planned, I realized now with sick horror. Perhaps over the sherry I had seen Vanessa and Mrs. Hacha drinking. Planned for just one purpose—my death by drowning!

My terror almost overwhelmed me. If this was planned, then there must be someone else down here on the beach. Someone ahead waiting to flash a light in the final gesture that would drive me into the water!

I glanced back. Someone carrying a flashlight was coming from the steps near the bathhouse. The light moved in leisurely fashion, searching the bathhouse and the cliff behind it. My first instinct was to run from that following light. But that was what they wanted me to do. For now I was sure that somewhere ahead in the darkness someone else waited. I stared out into the darkness and the fog, trying not to hear the ferocity of the tide. If I had to go into the sea, it would be on my terms, not Vanessa's.

Suppose I let the ebb tide take me, carry me out among those deadly reefs? If I could survive out there, the tide must turn soon. It must! I could swim back when the tide stopped running, *after* they thought I'd drowned. When they went back to the house . . . satisfied. But I couldn't swim in water like that in shirt and jeans. I began to pull them off where I stood, stripping to panties and bra.

Ahead, not far away, a light flashed!

"Samantha!" a low voice called. "It's me, *Adrian!* I have to talk to you! Please!"

Adrian was here. It was *Adrian* they planned to give me to the ebb tide! Adrian, the one among them I'd thought my friend. And I remembered that Adrian was the one among them I had most to fear in the turmoil of water I could hear out there. I had seen what Adrian could do in the sea. But Adrian did not know as much about my ability. My chance was there.

The fog swirled about me coldly. I shivered, steeling myself against cold water on my hot skin as I waded in silently, stealthily.

"Samantha?" his low voice called anxiously. "Answer me, please! Before they get here, I must talk to you!"

I began to feel the pull of the water, terribly strong. I let the ebb take me, barely moving arms and legs beneath water that seemed warming as I got used to it. I made fifty yards, sixty. Fog hid even the vague outline of the beach now.

His light flashed again back there, searching the beach, and as I looked back fearfully, I saw too that other flashlight, moving faster now, already almost to where I'd left my clothes.

"She's in the water! I've found her clothes!" a

man's voice shouted exultantly. Karl's, a hateful voice.

"I didn't see her!" Adrian's voice said.

"I'm going after her!" Karl said, dropping the flashlight. "You're not the only one who can swim, Hacha!"

"Stay where you are, unless you want to drown, you fool!" Adrian shouted. Adrian was coming after me. I heard him splash into deep water. I heard him dive and start swimming. Pricked by terror, I began to swim too, involuntarily, forgetting my plan to conserve my strength.

I had never moved through the water as fast in my life as I was now, propelled by the ebb tide and swimming hard with it. Already I was far from the beach, and I realized suddenly that I was being drawn inexorably toward the cliffs on the south side of the inlet—the one direction I'd meant to avoid, but pursued by Adrian, I had forgotten.

In panic now, I remembered the underwater caves, the natural tunnel leading in with a deadly maelstrom of spinning water above it on a tide like this. I was being sucked toward that vortex, to drown in the tunnel beneath. I turned away in terror, swimming raggedly as I tried in panic to fight my way at an angle away from that horrible place. Behind me I heard Adrian stop swimming to call to me.

"Samantha! Don't fight it! Let me help you!"

He seemed closer, *much closer*. Almost within reach of me, and all that I could think of was that he, *Adrian*, was part of the plot to drown me here in this awful place.

I turned away from him in terror: *"No!"* I cried *"No!"*

I began to swim again, desperately, but almost at once he was upon me. A hand reaching through the dark water caught my ankle, dragging me down. I kicked free, but we came up together. His arms caught me, and his strength was greater than mine. Sobbing for breath, I tried to fight him, to free myself. Only, as we fought, I began to hear what he was trying to tell me so desperately.

"This is the only way . . . I . . . can help you! You can stay alive! You can see Paul again! *But only with my help!*"

"I won't go into that awful place with you!" I panted. *"No!"*

"You must!" he hissed furiously. *"Listen to me!* Paul was coming here to see Vanessa, to demand to know where you are. But my mother told him Vanessa wasn't here. Paul phoned from Pescadero, and he could still be there! Stop fighting me! *It's almost too late!*"

It *was* too late. I could feel the vortex taking me, even as he dragged the mask over my face while I fought against it involuntarily. In that last desperate moment before we were both sucked under, I saw him tugging at his own snorkel mask.

He was trying to signal something that in my panic I did not understand. Then I felt the vortex take me. I screamed behind my mask. I was being spun around, sucked down . . . down . . .

I felt my body strike Adrian, and his hands take my shoulders, guiding me. I was being partly pushed, partly washed through the utter darkness. Rock bruised and grazed me in passing, and I knew I was in the tunnel. But the effort of swimming was not mine now, but his. Frozen in fear and shock, I could make no effort to help myself.

My panting, terrified breathing was using up the air in my mask too quickly, I sensed. I began to suffocate. I fought against it for as long as I could; then the primal impulses took over, and I screamed and tried to tear away the mask.

"Samantha, it's all right now!" a voice gasped in my ear. *"It's . . . all right!"*

I was breathing air again, I realized, my lungs pumping fresh, cold air that smelled of dampness and the sea. The mask was gone, and Adrian's arm was supporting me in the thick, terrifying darkness inside the cave. The water around us still swelled and receded from our swim through the tunnel, and each time it rose, I felt the rock face bump my bruised body.

"I thought . . . you'd drowned," he muttered. "But we got through. We're in the cave. You must help me now! Hold on to the rock!"

I grasped it instinctively and clung there. I felt him climb out of the water. His hands beneath my armpits began to lift me, to drag me from the swelling water over the rock floor of the cave. Rock grazed my thighs.

"We made it!" he muttered, as though he had thought it impossible. A light flashed,

showing me the sloping underwater cave that I feared, with its bands of colored rock, the dark water lapping at its floor.

I choked and couldn't tell him of my terror, of the claustrophobia that had nothing to do with the fear of drowning. He was urging me to my feet, moving me back from the swelling water that must rise higher as the tide changed.

"You'll be safe here," he muttered, flashing the light about the gloomy cave. "I'll tell her I lost you out there. I'll tell her I came in here but there was no sign of you, you must have been carried out to the reefs and drowned there."

I shuddered. "Adrian, please! I can't stay here alone!"

"You must!" he said grimly. He glanced around. "I'll have to go! They must be getting suspicious *now*! They'll guess I'm down here."

"*I can't!*" I quavered, thinking of the walls pressing in, the awful darkness when he had gone.

"There's no other way!" he said fiercely. "I've got to get up there, or they'll come down here searching for you. Vanessa and my mother both know the way in. They've been here before. My mother many times. They'll kill you if they find you still alive! *They have to kill you now!* Can't you realize that, and help me?"

"Will you . . . come back?"

"With Paul, if I can," he said.

"Paul?" I stared at him. He had tried to tell me something about Paul up there on the surface. Something about Pescadero? In my blind panic, I hadn't understood.

"I told you—Paul phoned from Pescadero," he said. "He was coming here to see his mother, to demand to know where you were. But my mother told him Mrs. Acton wasn't here. He could still be in Pescadero. . . ."

"But Paul doesn't know what's happening here!" I said, losing hope again.

"Listen," he said, "and try to understand! My mother locked Sara in her room, but while I waited for them to drive you to the cliff path, I let her out. I told her to phone her father and tell him what was happening here. I said he should bring Paul Acton with him. I told her to do that and then hide until they get here."

"Adrian, please! Wait till the tide turns, and take me with you. I can hide among the rocks, or on the beach!"

"*No!*" he said. "I've been gone too long. If they saw you with me, *alive* . . . His flashlight moved, showing me again the hole in the wall that led into the next cave. "Watch the water. If you see light coming, hide in the next cave. They won't look *there. I know this!*"

He thrust his flashlight and the second mask into my hand. "Remember, when I come back, it will be in darkness. Anyone with a flashlight is your enemy. *Hide from them!*"

He pulled down his mask, dived with barely a ripple, and was gone.

I crouched where he had left me, shivering and gripping the flashlight and the mask. Water rose and fell against the floor of the

cave, disturbed by his dive. Vanessa would not
have the courage to dive in here, I thought. But
Karl might. The thought of that man catching
me in this awful place was too much. I would
go mad. No padded cell of Finisterre could be
as horrible. I would die of terror. Even if he
came to Finisterre, Paul would never know
what had happened to me. Tears of self-pity
came welling, and I cried for a long time.

I was staring at the water through tears, and
there was light there. Light that grew slowly
stronger. Someone with a flashlight was in the
tunnel swimming toward me, and Adrian had
said anyone with a light was my enemy! I
struggled to my feet, danger driving me. My
light picked out the hole. He had said *she*
would not dare to look in there. I could reach
the hole quite easily, I found. I glanced back in
terror, keeping my own light away from the
water. Whoever was in the tunnel was close,
too close. I risked one quick glance down
through the hole, seeing a rock floor no more
than four feet below. I switched off the light
and climbed through.

I crouched in utter darkness with the mask
beside me on the rock floor, the light held like a
weapon in my hand, listening to water lapping
against rock as two swimmers approached.
They surfaced, and I heard their soft grunts of
relief as they dragged off their masks to breathe
gustily. *Women, two women!* I listened to
breathless voices I could barely hear above the
frightened drumbeat of my heart. Voices made
unrecognizable by their need for oxygen and

the effort of swimming. Lights flashed about.

"She's not here," a voice gasped. "But we had to check."

"Adrian told you that. The tide took her out among the reefs, and they'll never find her! You have nothing to fear from her *now*, I promise you."

I listened to the drip of water, the scrape of rubber wet suits on rock. Light lanced through the opening above my head, and I crouched lower instinctively.

"She could be in there!" It was Vanessa's voice. But in this place, in these circumstances, this seemed too horrible for me to accept.

"In the dark? Forced into the water naked and leaving her clothes on the beach?"

I couldn't mistake Mrs. Hacha's contemptuous laugh. "How could she *see* that opening in the darkness in here? Or know what was on the other side of it? If she had gotten out of the tunnel alive, she'd still be sitting right here on the rock floor, not daring to move. But I don't trust Adrian anymore. So we will check. My son has changed. That girl did this to him, the one I told you I had to get rid of. We have to protect our sons from women like these."

"I didn't want Samantha hurt," Vanessa protested uneasily. "I told you that, Catherine. I wanted them kept apart. That was all. Men forget quickly, and as you said, we must protect our sons."

"You're weak, Vanessa," Catherine Hacha said. "I wouldn't be surprised if Karl decided you should be locked up again for your own protection. As he had to decide once before. He's still a doctor, you know. *Your doctor.* Or have you conveniently forgotten that? Here, take my light and look in the other cave. Perhaps you'll feel better tomorrow, with all this over and done with."

"*I couldn't!*" Vanessa said in a terrified voice. "*He's still in there!* You know that."

"You didn't want *him* hurt either, remember?" Catherine Hacha's voice reminded her. "But did you cry when he died, Vanessa? Or did you take his wealth, *all of it,* for yourself, including his son's share? *And* enjoy it?"

"You know it wasn't like that!" Vanessa cried.

"I know exactly how it was, Vanessa. I was there, remember?" Mrs. Hacha said coldly. "Take the light and look in there and tell me what you see. Are you afraid of the dead? Fear always was a part of your particular psychosis, wasn't it, Vanessa? Karl may consider this recurring fear of yours dangerous to the rest of us."

"*No!* You wouldn't do that!"

"Then do as I say. You will not see that stupid girl who aroused your jealousy in there. She's dead. Drowned. Her body's caught in the kelp out there somewhere where nobody will ever find it. Take the flashlight!"

Light flooded through the hole above me, light that trembled in a nervous hand. I was about to be discovered, murdered perhaps. But in my growing anger at the things I had heard, that didn't seem to matter anymore. My hair matted from the dive, my eyes staring furiously, I reared up into the beam of bright light.

"Vanessa!" I screamed. "*What have you done to me, Vanessa?*"

Momentarily I was looking into Vanessa Acton's dark eyes close to mine—eyes grown unnaturally large and staring wildly back at me from a face growing ashen pale from the horror twisting it. Then she shrieked and fell backward, dropping her flashlight with the sound of shattering glass. Utter darkness blinded me, filling both caves. Vanessa was shrieking frantically as she groped for the broken flashlight.

Another, hoarser voice cried in horror, "You fool! You've broken my mask!"

As terrified as they were now, I listened to the sounds of hysterical fear as I groped, sobbing, for my flashlight. I heard their shrieks as they heard me moving, and their terror grew. I heard one dive in terror into the water, then the other.

It grew quiet. The lapping water stilled. My shaking hand found the flashlight that had rolled beyond my reach. I got up weakly and switched it on, inexpressibly grateful for its brightness. Out there, as I peered fearfully through the hole, the cave was empty, except for a shattered snorkel mask lying near the water.

One of them had no mask, no air. Then I saw the strap of the other mask. Perhaps both masks were useless. I remembered what Adrian had told me about it being impossible to swim into the cave without a mask. Shivering, I found my own mask still unharmed, and picked it up.

It was my key to freedom. I started to scramble through into the outer cave, but curiosity prompted me to check first this other cave that had proved my salvation. Turning, I swung the light in an arc, revealing a great cavern, larger than the other, with a flat rock thrusting up in the center. A rock with . . .

The flashlight steadied, and I screamed. The naked body of a girl with jet-black hair lay on her back upon the tablelike rock. Her eyes were open and staring. Her face had the waxen pallor of death, and there was a ghastly wound in her head. Around her neck a gold cross hung pitifully from a chain. *The cross Adrian had given the girl he loved, Jane Buchan!*

I saw the other deflated figure lying horribly beside her, a caricature of a tall man with hair that once had been blond. The body was encased in shrunken, parchmentlike skin that covered it to the gaping mouth, the empty eye sockets, the seaweed hair.

Shrieking, I scrambled through into the outer cave. I fell into the water, losing both light and mask but barely noticing the loss in my frenzy to escape from that horrible cavern. I would have tried to escape without mask or light, and surely drowned, only, as I swam down toward the tunnel's exit, light blazed at me through the water, and a new and greater fear stopped me abruptly.

It was as though Adrian's voice warned me again, even through my abject terror. "*Anyone with a flashlight is your enemy. Hide from them!"*

I was trying to turn back, even knowing the people behind the lights must see the bubbles, the swirling water. I knew the instant when they saw and came after me fast, two figures in wet suits. No snorkels this time, but Aqualungs. There was no way of escape from them now, I knew, even as I swam from them with the desperation of despair. There was nowhere left to escape *to*, except those horrible caverns that must soon hold another body, for they had no other outlet save this underwater tunnel from which I swam.

I surfaced, gasping, inside the outer cave. I scrambled out, with the flashlights following faster than I could swim. I glanced back in terror as I climbed through the hole into the other cavern. A dark head bobbed from the water. The flashlight jerked about as the swimmer tore at the face mask.

"Samantha!"

The gasping voice, barely heard above the pounding of my terrified heart, my panting breath, meant nothing to me. I fled from the sound and the pursuer.

In the darkness, my hands reaching out touched firm cold flesh that I recoiled from involuntarily. *Jane Buchan's body!* And suddenly, there was nowhere to go. My back was against the wall of rock, and I stayed there, my legs barely supporting me while I watched the first flashlight probe through the hole into the cavern. I watched the first seallike black head appear in the light. The flashlight swung, probing. It steadied on the bodies lying side by side, and a man's shocked voice said, *"My God! Look there!"*

But the other torch had found *me*. I closed my eyes against the glare, with my knees starting to sag as the man behind it cried, *"There she is!"*

The light danced as he came toward me fast, and it was too late for flight, even if I'd had the strength. Strong hands seized me, and I was past resistance. But unbelievingly then, the same hands became gentle, were holding me close, while a voice I listened to incredulously was saying, *"Samantha!* Oh, my God! *What have they done to you?"* Paul's voice, Paul's arms.

"Oh, Paul, *Paul!"* I cried as the tears began to flow, and I just seemed to keep on saying that over and over while he held me and kissed me until the other man came over.

"Don't let her see!" he said warningly, and I felt Paul nod.

But I *had* seen, and I was remembering Catherine Hacha, and Vanessa, and that thing on the stone slab was what they had been talking about. *It was Paul's father, whose body never had been found.*

I tried to tell Paul that, but Paul silenced me. "We'll swim her out between us, and I'll share my air with her, Sergeant Sheridan," he said. "Help me with her. Other things can wait. I just want her out of here!"

Of the swim back I remember only Paul's

arms holding me, the tube from his Aqua-lung feeding me oxygenated air before we rose into a world beneath a canopy of stars. But not much more than that, until I wakened in the bedroom I'd been given in Finisterre. Paul was dozing in a chair beside my bed. He stirred as though he sensed my waking and opened his eyes and said anxiously, "Samantha?"

"I love you, Paul," I said.

He nodded. "It was because I know that, Samantha, that I refused to believe Vanessa," he said grimly. "She gave me back the ring I bought you. She said you didn't want to go through with our marriage. She said you had gone to New York to live, and you were not coming back."

I smiled. Manlike, he hadn't even noticed that I still wore his ring. "She lied," I said gently, and showed him the real ring. "She asked me where you bought it, and I told her."

"And she ordered a replica," he said. "Only afterward she kept avoiding me. I wanted to know where you were, Samantha. If it was all over, I needed to hear that from you. I meant to come here tonight to ask Vanessa about that, because the chauffeur at Bel Air said she was coming to Finisterre tonight. I'd finished the job in Phoenix, so drove through to Pescadero. I phoned Finisterre from there, but Mrs. Hacha said Vanessa wasn't here and wasn't coming here this week, to her knowledge. I saw no reason to come here after what she said, but I was too tired to drive back to Los Angeles, so I stayed in Pescadero."

"She lied, too."

"I know that now. The man in the water with us last night was Sara Sheridan's father. Sara phoned him and said he should contact me, because Adrian Hacha said I might still be in Pescadero. Her father told me Sara was scared. She said she had been locked in her room, and she thought you were being murdered. Until Sergeant Sheridan told me that, I had no idea you could possibly be at Finisterre. We both owe Sara plenty, and I mean to repay her for that when . . ." He broke off, frowning.

"When what, darling?"

"Samantha, remember what you told Sergeant Sheridan and me last night about Vanessa and Mrs. Hacha losing their masks in the cavern?"

I shook my head, only vaguely remembering their questions. "I remember that Vanessa broke Mrs. Hacha's mask. I remember seeing the strap of Vanessa's mask on the cave floor."

"Vanessa drowned last night," he said. "So did Mrs. Hacha. They recovered the bodies this morning out near the reefs. That was what I meant about repaying Sara Sheridan for us last night. With Vanessa's death, my father's estate goes to me, I believe."

"*I* want to thank Adrian," I said. "Without Adrian's help, I would have drowned last night, as Vanessa and his mother did. I would have been sucked down into that horrible place, and I had no mask, either."

It was then that Paul told me Adrian had been arrested last night on his own confession as an accessory to murder and attempted murder. For Adrian had confessed that his mother, by persuading Paul's father to swim on an ebb tide, was responsible for his death. Adrian found the body in the cavern, but could not bring himself to tell the police and implicate his mother. Adrian was sure Vanessa had a part in that too, and she *was* the one who benefited most from Paul's father's death. But Vanessa couldn't answer that charge now. Neither could Catherine Hacha.

But when Mrs. Hacha murdered Jane Buchan, and forced her son to burn the evidence of her clothes left behind in the dressing-room on the beach, that was too much for poor Adrian. Jane was dead, but when they planned to kill me too, he rebelled and turned against his mother and Vanessa.

And as police probing continued, we learned, Paul and I, that Vanessa had been a patient at Finisterre for almost two years while Paul, working hard at Stanford, thought her vacationing in Europe, because Paul's father did not want him to know that Vanessa was a schizophrenic. Vanessa fell under the influence of Catherine Hacha, the head nurse, while a patient at Finisterre. From then on, the strong-willed, vicious woman dominated Vanessa as she did Adrian. It was Mrs. Hacha who influenced the purchase of Finisterre and its library, and her own installation as its virtual mistress.

But we do not live in Finisterre, and never will. For we are married now and still in love, and Finisterre, we both agree, is no place to bring up our children.

More Gothics from SIGNET